Slimming Magazine

BUSINESSMAN'S
CALORIE COUNTER

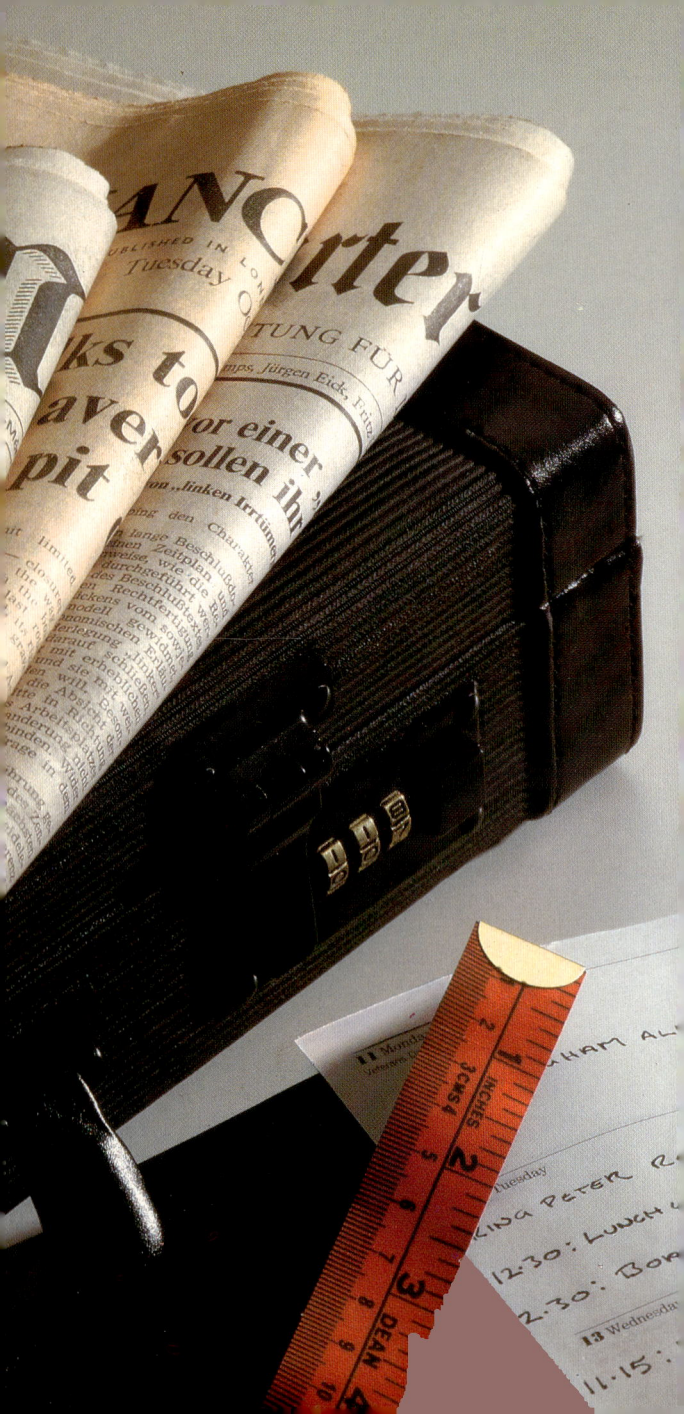

Slimming Magazine

BUSINESSMAN'S CALORIE COUNTER

OCTOPUS BOOKS

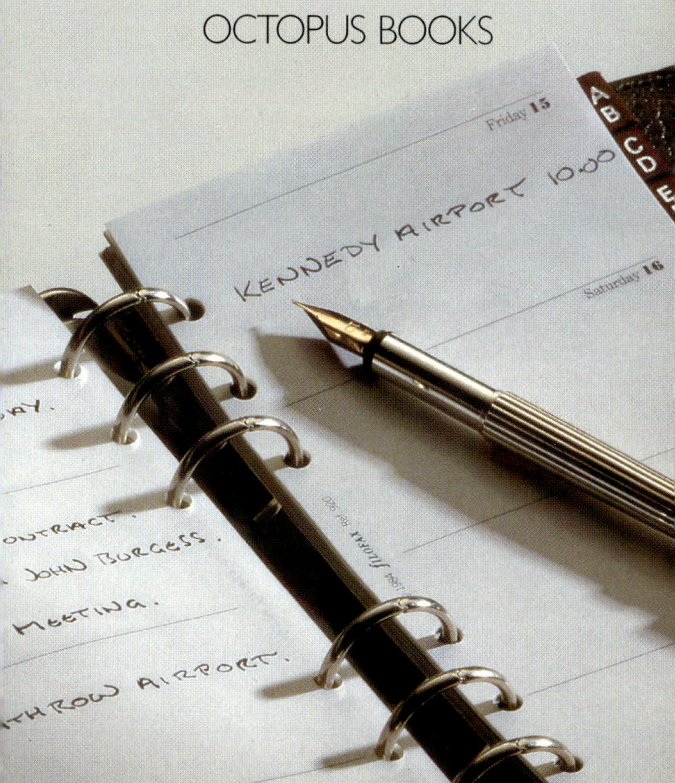

First published 1985 by
Octopus Books Limited
59 Grosvenor Street
London W1

© Text: Slimming Magazine Publications Limited 1985
© Photographs: Octopus Books Limited 1985

ISBN 0 7064 2321 6

Produced by Mandarin Publishers Limited
22a Westlands Road
Quarry Bay, Hong Kong

Printed in Hong Kong

Editors: Sybil Greatbatch and Glynis McGuinness
Nutritionist: Dr Nigel Dickie

CONTENTS

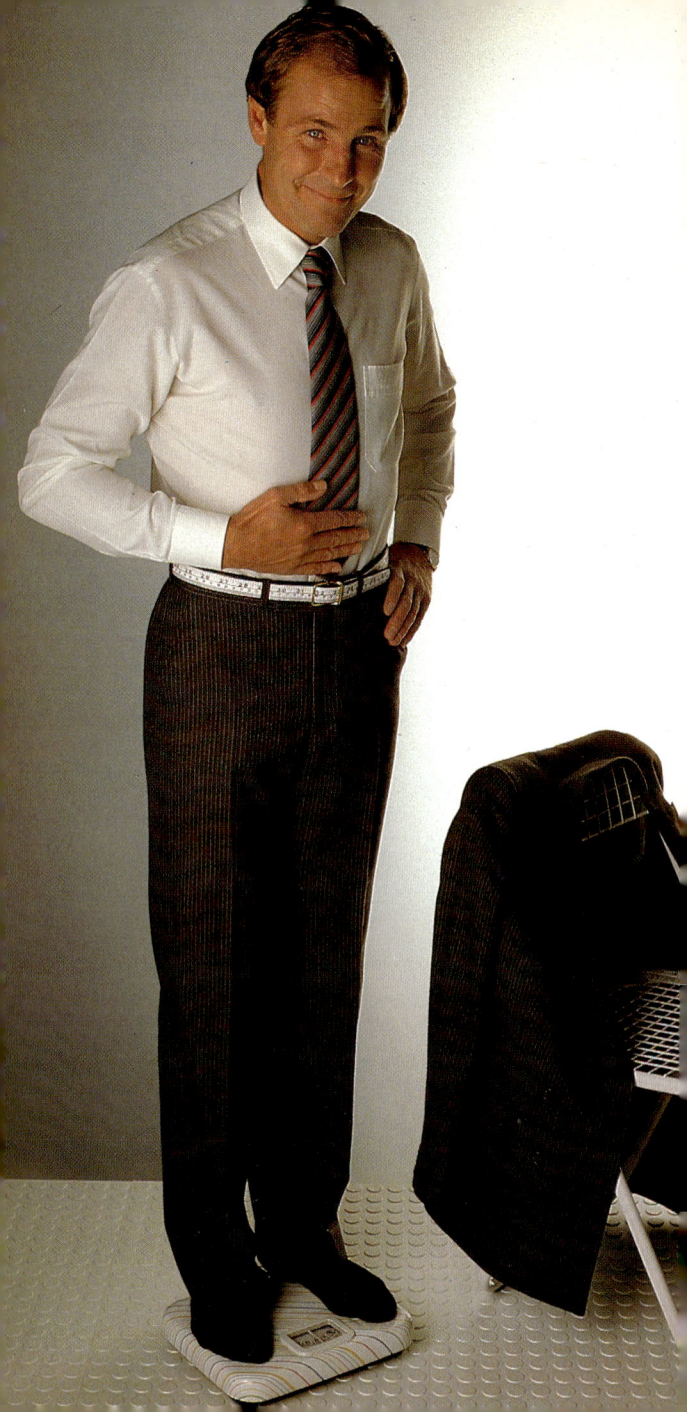

INTRODUCTION

Until quite recently, a man often had to be frightened into dieting. Usually it was his doctor, his insurance broker or some first tell-tale signs of ill health that started him on a weight loss campaign. But today, men as well as women embark on diets to improve their appearance as well as their health.

When men do make up their minds to slim, they are often more successful than women. This is partly because men can consume a higher number of calories a day, so they do not need to diet quite so strictly — or, if they do diet strictly, they lose weight faster. Also, men who are at work all day do not have to face the same constant temptations to nibble that the housewife does.

Men are more likely than women to turn to exercise as a solution to weight problems. But while gradually increasing one's physical activity is a good idea for all of us, the man who thinks that he is going to peel off a couple of stone by going to a gym two or three times a week is in for a disappointment. If he doesn't diet at the same time, it is unlikely to do anything worthwhile for his weight. Certainly regular exercise can play an important part in controlling weight, but irregular exercise alone is likely to produce a disappointingly slow weight reduction and sudden *strenuous* exercise can be downright dangerous.

However, an overweight man who takes the right kind of exercise is less likely to suffer from a coronary heart attack than an overweight man who doesn't exercise at all. This is because exercise improves the coronary circulation, and may have an affect on the way the body handles cholesterol and fat.

Although this may surprise you, strenuous exercise does not do nearly as much good as you might imagine. About an hour's walking each day would be very much more effective both in terms of burning up calories and in improving coronary

11

circulation. It is important that you do this every day, so try to build some extra walking into your daily routine. Can you walk to the station and back instead of taking your car, or park your car a good 15 minutes away from the office and walk the remaining distance? It doesn't matter if the daily walk is divided up into three or four 15-minute walks, it will still have the same benefit.

How much do you need to lose?

Check the chart on page 14 to calculate your ideal weight. The figures are for a medium-frame figure and your personal ideal could be about 5 kg/10 lb or so either side of these weights. Your best plan is to aim for the medium-frame figure and see what you feel like at that weight. If you think you could go a little lower, continue dieting. If you feel too skinny, you can allow a few pounds to creep back on. Heights are minus footwear and weights include an allowance of 1 kg/2 to 3 lb for light indoor clothing.

Weigh yourself once a week, at the same time of day, wearing similar clothes. Because of fluctuations of water in the body you are likely to be lighter first thing in the morning than in the evening.

A man who has been over-indulging for some time will probably see a massive weight loss during the first week. This will partly be the body getting rid of excess water. As dieting progresses, a man should settle down to a steady weight loss of about 1 kg/2 to 3 lb a week.

How to plan your diet

Every successful slimming diet you have ever tried or heard of has only one real secret: it is low in calories. There are no special foods, such as grapefruit or pineapples, that will magically make the pounds disappear. The calorie total of what you eat a day is what counts. No way has yet been found to change the prime physical law that if you eat more calories than your body needs, it will store

RIGHT: Walking is an effective form of exercise; build a 15-minute walk into your journey to and from work.

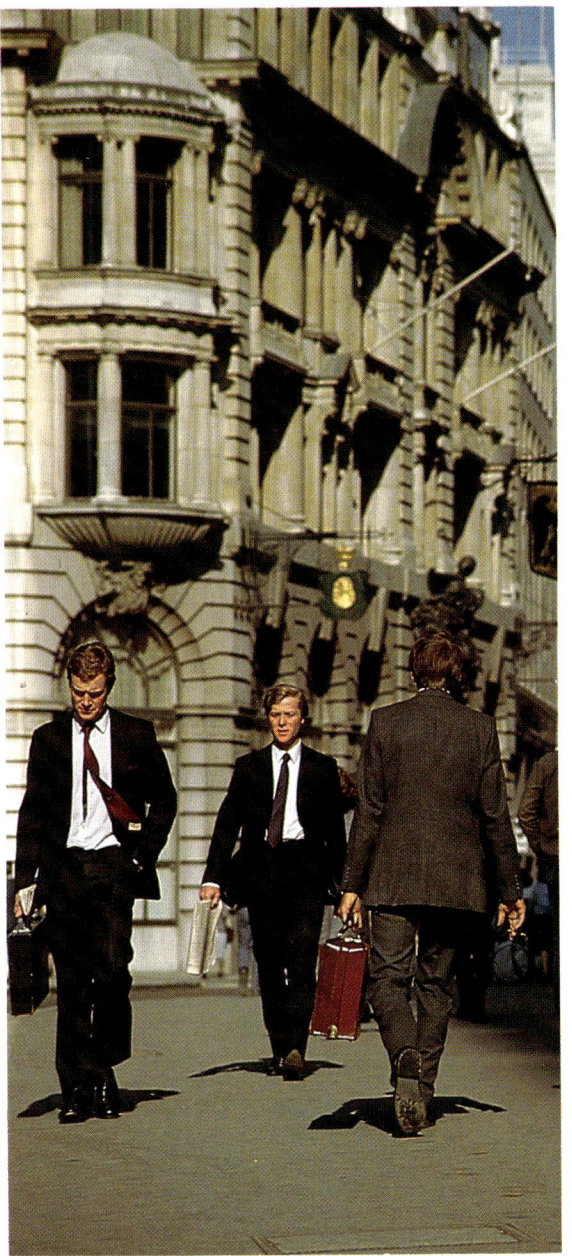

them as fat; and if you eat fewer calories than your body burns up in energy, it will call on its fat reserves to make up the necessary difference and you will get slim.

Generally, the more overweight you are, the more rapidly you will lose weight when you start dieting. As you near your target weight, you may need to restrict your calories a little more to rid yourself of all your surplus.

Good health depends as much on what you eat as how many calories you consume. The first rule of good nutrition is variety. Each food provides a different combination of the nutrients your body

1.55 m	(5-ft-1)	56 kg	(123 lb or 8-st-11)
1.57 m	(5-ft-2)	57.5 kg	(127 lb or 9-st-1)
1.60 m	(5-ft-3)	59 kg	(130 lb or 9-st-4)
1.63 m	(5-ft-4)	60.5 kg	(133 lb or 9-st-7)
1.65 m	(5-ft-5)	62 kg	(136 lb or 9-st-10)
1.68 m	(5-ft-6)	64 kg	(141 lb or 10-st-1)
1.70 m	(5-ft-7)	66 kg	(145 lb or 10-st-5)
1.73 m	(5-ft-8)	67.5 kg	(149 lb or 10-st-9)
1.75 m	(5-ft-9)	69.5 kg	(153 lb or 10-st-13)
1.78 m	(5-ft-10)	72 kg	(158 lb or 11-st-4)
1.80 m	(5-ft-11)	73.5 kg	(162 lb or 11-st-8)
1.83 m	(6-ft-0)	75.5 kg	(166 lb or 11-st-12)
1.85 m	(6-ft-1)	77.5 kg	(171 lb or 12-st-3)
1.88 m	(6-ft-2)	80 kg	(176 lb or 12-st-8)
1.90 m	(6-ft-3)	82.5 kg	(182 lb or 13-st-0)

needs. If you vary the content of your meals as much as possible, you should automatically obtain all the nutrients necessary for good health.

Setting your calorie allowance

If you have more than 20 kg/3 st to lose, it should not be necessary to reduce your calories below 1,750 a day. If you have just 6 to 7 kg/1 st to lose, set your allowance at 1,250. Between about 7 kg/1 st and 20 kg/3 st excess, aim for 1,500 Calories a day.

You can, if you prefer, think in terms of your weekly calorie total. This means that if you have a business lunch one day, you can allow yourself extra calories, then cut back the following day. Your diet will be more successful if you plan in advance what you are going to eat. If you know you will be visiting a wine bar at lunchtime, for example, work out how many glasses of wine you can 'afford', and the lowest calorie food choice. If you eat and drink first, then calculate the damage, you could be in for a shock.

Dieting rules

● Set your daily calorie allowance between 1,250 and 1,750.
● Include a wide variety of foods in your daily menus to ensure you get all the nutrients you need for good health.
● Weigh and measure all foods accurately. The only exceptions are leafy green vegetables, lettuce, cucumber and cress, which are so low in calories you can pile them on your plate.
● If you exceed your calorie allowance in one day, do not despair and give up. Make up for the excess the next day by eating less. You will lose exactly the same amount of weight by eating 2,000 Calories one day and 1,000 the next as eating 1,500 Calories each day.
● Some drinks are calorie-free: water, black tea and coffee (without sugar). These can be consumed in unlimited amounts. However, most drinks contain calories and some are very high. Remember to include all calorie-containing drinks in your daily total. Alcoholic drinks are listed on pages 79–89, non-alcoholic drinks on pages 91–95.

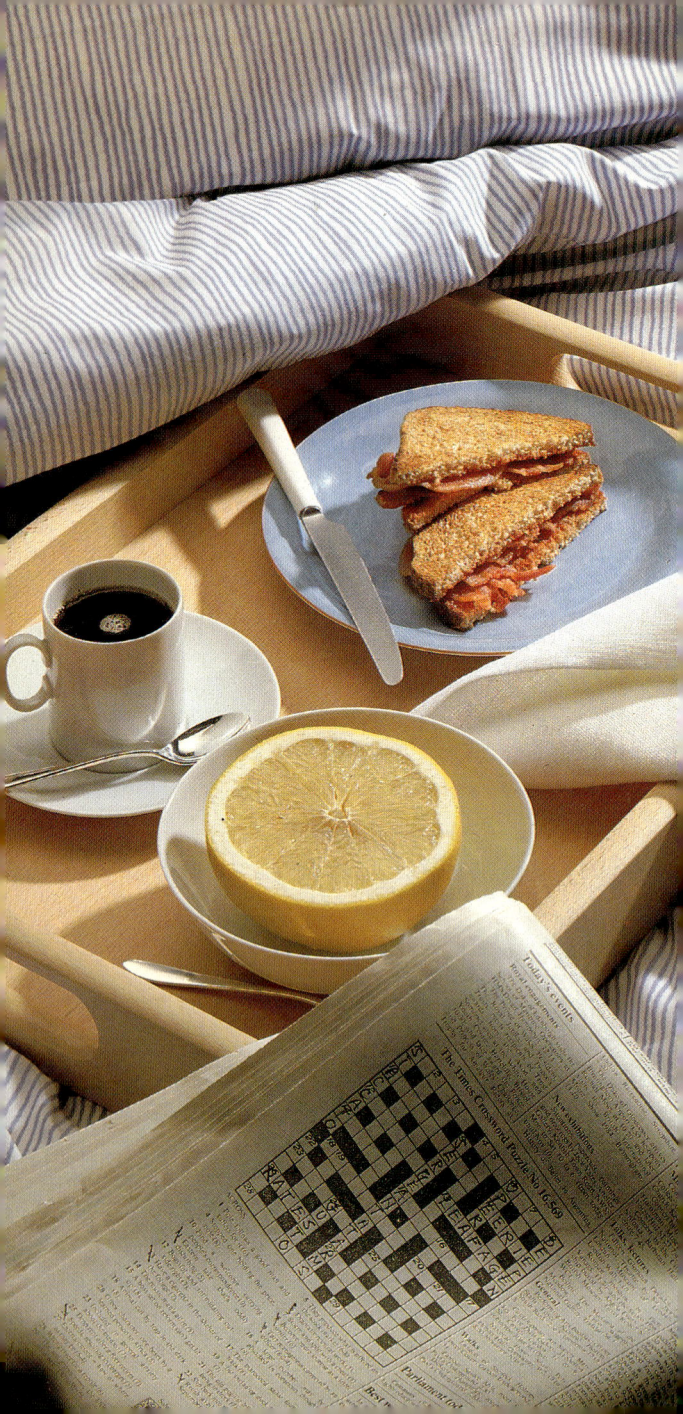

BREAKFASTS

Calculate your breakfast calories from the charts below or select one of the calorie-counted recipes on pages 24–27. Most people find it fairly easy not to eat very much at breakfast time, and many people are happy to miss breakfast entirely. If you would prefer to save calories for later in the day, there is absolutely no reason why you shouldn't miss breakfast, unless this encourages you to buy a sticky bun on the way to work! If you ever have to breakfast away from home, look up average calorie counts for hotel servings in the chart.

If you have breakfast at work, see Canteen Meals, page 33.

———————— Calorie cutters ————————

★ Substitute low-fat spread for butter or margarine on your breakfast toast and save 105 Calories per 25 g/1 oz.
* If you switch from Silver Top milk to skimmed, you will save 180 Calories for each 568 ml/1 pint. But if you find skimmed milk's less creamy taste a little difficult to take at first, try semi-skimmed milk, which will save you about 80 Calories.

Eggs

All the figures below are for medium-sized eggs. For large eggs, add 15 Calories; for small eggs, subtract 10 Calories

Boiled or poached, each	80
Fried, each	100
Scrambled, 1 egg scrambled with 15 ml/ 1 tablespoon skimmed milk	85
Scrambled, 1 egg scrambled with 5 ml/1 level teaspoon butter and 15 ml/1 tablespoon skimmed milk	120
Scrambled, average portion served in a hotel	250

17

Fish

Kedgeree, average restaurant portion	360
Kippers, boil-in-the-bag, 1 × 200 g/7 oz packet	370
Kippers, 1 whole medium, 175 g/6 oz	280
Smoked haddock, boil-in-the-bag, 1 × 198 g/7 oz packet	185
Smoked haddock fillet, poached, average portion, 125 g/4 oz	116

Meat

Bacon, 1 back rasher, well grilled or fried	80
Bacon, 1 streaky rasher, well grilled or fried	50
Black pudding, 50 g/2 oz raw weight, sliced and fried	170
Breakfast sausage, 50 g/2 oz	150
Ham, cooked, lean only, 25 g/1 oz	45
Kidneys, lamb's, grilled without fat, each	50
Kidneys, lamb's, fried, each	65
Sausage, beef, 1 large, well grilled	120
Sausage, beef, 1 chipolata, well grilled	50
Sausage, pork, 1 chipolata, well grilled	65
Sausage, pork, 1 large, well grilled	125
Sausage, pork and beef, 1 chipolata, well grilled	60
Sausage, pork and beef, 1 large, well grilled	125

Vegetables and spaghetti

Baked beans, 1 × 150 g/5 oz can	110
Baked beans, 1 × 225 g/8 oz can	160
Baked beans, per average canteen/restaurant portion	60
Mushrooms, all types, boiled, 50 g/2 oz raw weight	10
Mushrooms, flat, fried, 50 g/2 oz raw weight	100
Potatoes, sautéed, 125 g/4 oz	160
Spaghetti, canned in tomato sauce, 1 × 215g/7½ oz can	145
Tomatoes, grilled without fat, each	10
Tomatoes, fried, each	40

Fruit juices

Per small 150 ml/¼ pint glass:
Apple, unsweetened	50
Grapefruit, sweetened	55
Grapefruit, unsweetened	45
Orange, sweetened	75
Orange, unsweetened	55
Pineapple, unsweetened	75

Grapefruit

Canned, in natural juice, 150 g/5 oz	55
Canned, in syrup, 150 g/5 oz	85
Fresh, ½ medium	20

Cereals

All the following are average bowl servings:
All Bran, 40 g/1½ oz	105
All Bran, per individual box	105
Alpen, 25 g/1 oz	105
30% Bran Flakes, 25 g/1 oz	85
30% Bran Flakes, per individual box	85
Cornflakes, 25 g/1 oz	100
Cornflakes, per individual box	60
Porridge, made with 40 g/1½ oz rolled oats and water	175
Porridge, made with 25 g/1 oz instant porridge oats (e.g. Ready Brek) and 150 ml/¼ pint skimmed milk	160
Puffed Wheat, 25 g/1 oz	100
Rice Krispies, 25 g/1 oz	100
Rice Krispies, per individual box	75
Shredded Wheat, each	75
Special K, 25 g/1 oz	100
Special K, per individual box	60
Sultana Bran, 40 g/1½ oz	130
Weetabix, 2 biscuits	130

Additions to cereals:

If you add dried or fresh fruit to your cereal you probably won't need sugar. But if you decide you must indulge, each *rounded* teaspoon of sugar will cost you 35 Calories.

Apple, I medium	50
Apricots, dried, each	10
Banana, I small	50
Banana, I medium	80
Banana, I large	95
Bananas, dried, 15 g/½ oz	70
Dates, dried, stoned, 15 g/½ oz	35
Figs, dried, each	30
Grapes, black, 50 g/2 oz	30
Grapes, white, 50 g/2 oz	35
Nectarines, I medium	50
Peaches, I medium	35
Raisins, 15 ml/I level tablespoon	25
Strawberries, 50 g/2 oz	15
Sugar, 10 ml/I rounded teaspoon	35

Milk, milk substitutes and yogurt

Coffee creamer (e.g. Coffee-Mate), 10 ml/ I rounded teaspoon	15
Coffee creamer (e.g. Coffee-Mate), individual catering sachet	20
Full-fat milk (e.g. Silver Top), 25 ml/I fl oz	20
Full-fat milk (e.g. Silver Top), individual catering carton	10
Half cream, 15 ml/I tablespoon	20
Half cream, individual catering carton	20
Semi-skimmed milk, 25 ml/I fl oz	15
Single cream, 15 ml/I tablespoon	30
Single cream, individual catering carton	30
Skimmed milk, 25 ml/I fl oz	10
Skimmed milk powder, 10 ml/I rounded teaspoon	10
Skimmed milk powder, individual catering sachet	10
Yogurt, low-fat, natural, I × 150 g/5 oz carton	100
Yogurt, low-fat, fruit, I × 150 g/5 oz carton	140

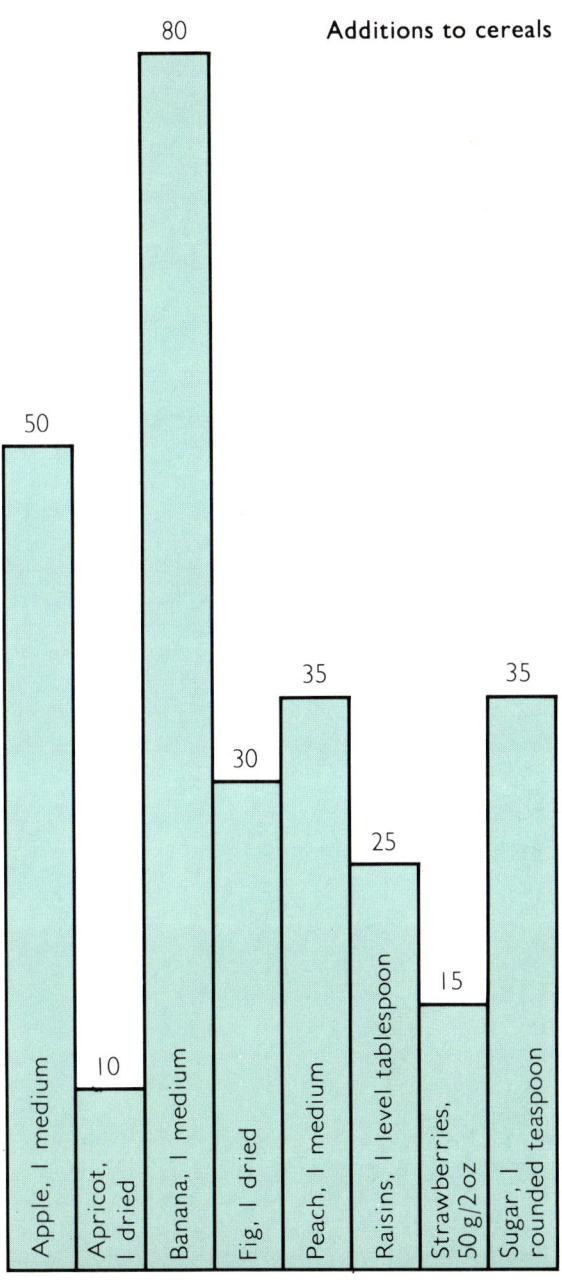

Additions to cereals

80

50

35

30

35

25

15

10

Apple, 1 medium

Apricot, 1 dried

Banana, 1 medium

Fig, 1 dried

Peach, 1 medium

Raisins, 1 level tablespoon

Strawberries, 50 g/2 oz

Sugar, 1 rounded teaspoon

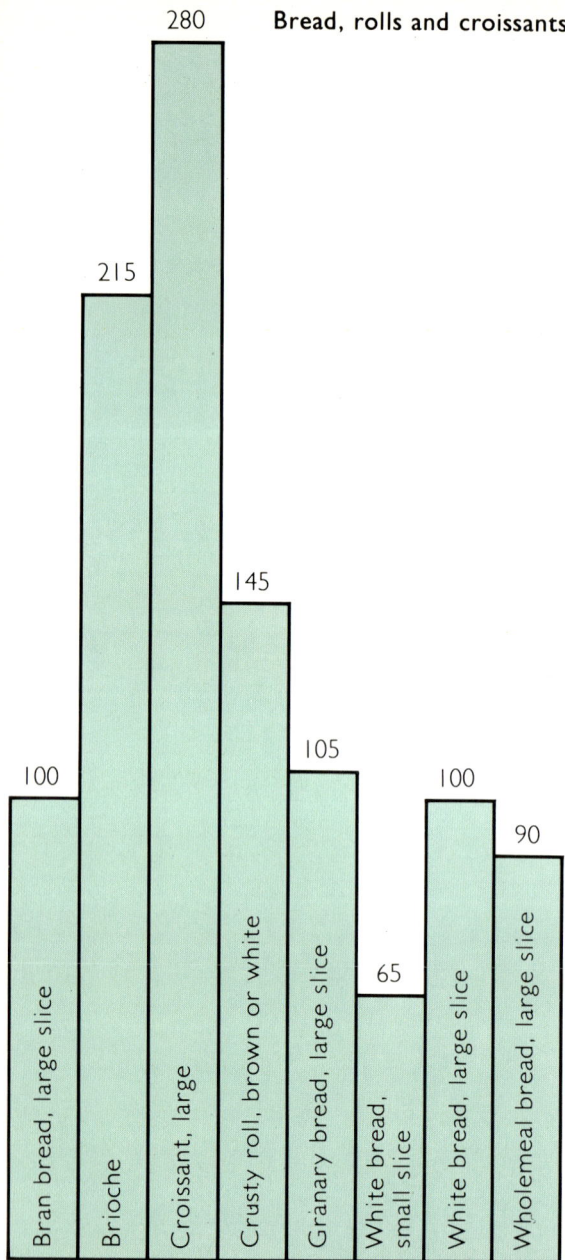

Bread, rolls and croissants

280 — Croissant, large

215 — Brioche

145 — Crusty roll, brown or white

105 — Granary bread, large slice

100 — Bran bread, large slice

100 — White bread, large slice

90 — Wholemeal bread, large slice

65 — White bread, small slice

Bread, croissants, rolls

Toast any of the following if you wish – calories will remain the same.

Aberdeen morning roll, 1 medium	185
Bagel, 1 medium, 40 g/1½ oz	150
Bap, 1 medium, 40 g/1½ oz	130
Bran bread, 1 small slice, 25 g/1 oz	65
Bran bread, 1 large slice, 40 g/1½ oz	100
Brioche roll, 1 medium, 45 g/1¾ oz	215
Brown bread, 1 small slice, 25 g/1 oz	65
Brown bread, 1 large slice, 40 g/1½ oz	95
Brown crusty roll, 1 medium, 45 g/1¾ oz	145
Brown soft roll, 1 medium, 45 g/1¾ oz	140
Cholla bread or Enriched bread, 1 × 40 g/1½ oz slice	165
Croissant, 1 small	165
Croissant, 1 large	280
Fried bread, 1 × 25 g/1 oz slice, unfried weight	160
Granary bread, 1 × 25 g/1 oz slice	70
Granary bread, 1 × 40 g/1½ oz slice	105
White bread, 1 × 25 g/1 oz slice	65
White bread, 1 × 40 g/1½ oz slice	100
White crusty roll, 45 g/1¾ oz	145
White soft roll, 45 g/1¾ oz	150
Wholemeal bread, 1 × 25 g/1 oz slice	60
Wholemeal bread, 1 × 40 g/1½ oz slice	90
Wholemeal roll, 45 g/1¾ oz	125

Butter and spreads

Butter, 5 ml/1 level teaspoon	35
Butter, individual catering pack	80
Cheese spread, 5 ml/1 level teaspoon	20
Cheese spread, per triangle	40
Honey, 5 ml/1 level teaspoon	20
Honey, clear, individual catering pack	60
Honey, set, individual catering pack	70
Jam, 5 ml/1 level teaspoon	15
Jam, individual catering pack	55
Lemon curd, 5 ml/1 level teaspoon	15
Low-fat spread, 5 ml/1 level teaspoon	15
Margarine, 5 ml/1 level teaspoon	35
Marmalade, 5 ml/1 level teaspoon	15
Marmalade, individual catering pack	55

Breakfast menus

All these menus are for single servings.

Fruit juice, toast and marmalade
250 Calories

Start with 120 ml/4 fl oz unsweetened apple, grape-fruit or orange juice. To follow, have 2 × 25 g/1 oz slices wholemeal bread, toasted, with 15 ml/1 level tablespoon low-fat spread and 15 ml/1 level table-spoon jam or marmalade.

Toast and Marmite or Bovril
250 Calories

Have 2 × 40 g/1½ oz slices wholemeal bread, toast-ed, with 15 ml/1 level tablespoon low-fat spread and 10 ml/2 level teaspoons Marmite or Bovril.

Grapefruit plus bacon sandwich
250 Calories

Start with ½ grapefruit. Follow with a sandwich made from 2 × 25 g/1 oz slices wholemeal bread, filled with 2 grilled streaky rashers bacon and 15 ml/1 level tablespoon tomato ketchup.

Fruit juice plus All Bran and raisins
250 Calories

Start with 120 ml/4 fl oz unsweetened apple, grape-fruit or orange juice. To follow, place 50 g/2 oz All Bran in an individual serving bowl. Stir in 15 ml/1 level tablespoon raisins or sultanas. Serve with 120 ml/4 fl oz skimmed milk.

Cornflakes plus toast
250 Calories

Place 25 g/1 oz cornflakes in an individual serving bowl. Serve with 120 ml/4 fl oz skimmed milk and 10 ml/1 rounded teaspoon sugar. To follow, have 1 × 25 g/1 oz slice wholemeal toast with 5 ml/1 level teaspoon low-fat spread.

Fruit juice plus porridge
250 Calories

Start with 150 ml/¼ pint unsweetened apple, grape-fruit or orange juice. To follow, serve porridge made from 25 g/1 oz porridge oats or hot oat cereal and 150 ml/¼ pint skimmed milk. (Follow packet instructions.) Serve with 10 ml/1 rounded teaspoon honey or sugar.

Weetabix and banana
250 Calories

Place 2 Weetabix in an individual serving bowl. Stir in 1 medium banana, sliced. Serve with 120 ml/4 fl oz skimmed milk.

Muesli
250 Calories

Place 50 g/2 oz muesli in an individual serving bowl. Serve with 120 ml/4 fl oz skimmed milk.

Shredded Wheat
250 Calories

Place 2 Shredded Wheat in an individual serving bowl. Serve with 150 ml/¼ pint skimmed milk and 10 ml/1 rounded teaspoon sugar.

Calorie cutters

★ Mushrooms are very low in calories if you poach them in water, but do not fry them with your bacon or sausage. If you do, they will absorb all the fat from the meat.
★ Some cereals are much heavier than others. If you want to fill your breakfast bowl, choose a light cereal such as corn-flakes or Puffed Wheat.

Fruit juice plus poached egg on toast
250 Calories

Start with 150 ml/$\frac{1}{4}$ pint unsweetened apple, grape-fruit or orange juice. To follow, poach 1 size 3 egg and serve on 1 × 40 g/1$\frac{1}{2}$ oz slice wholemeal toast, topped with 10 ml/2 level teaspoons low-fat spread.

Sausages and baked beans
250 Calories

Grill 2 pork or beef chipolata sausages well.

BELOW: Fruit juice plus poached egg on toast.

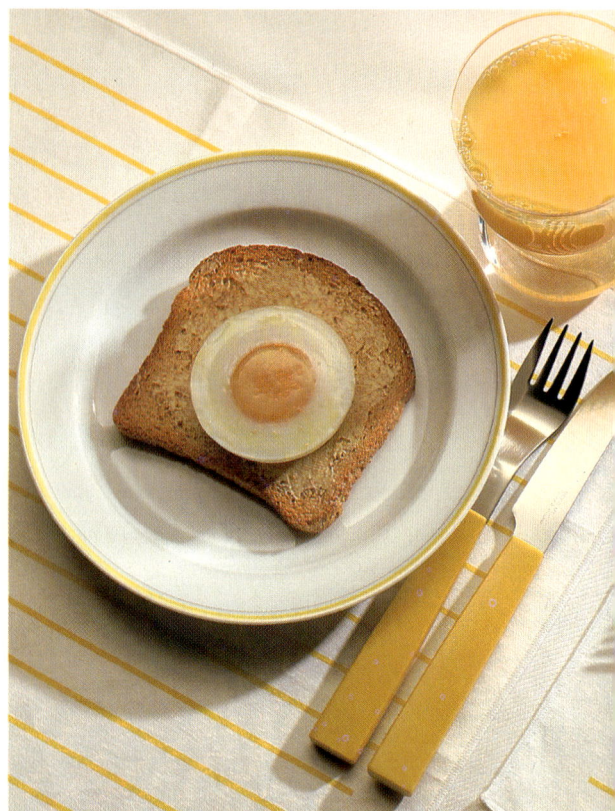

Meanwhile, heat 1 × 150 g/5.3 oz can baked beans in tomato sauce. Serve with the sausages.

Scrambled egg and bacon
250 Calories

In a non-stick pan, scramble 1 size 3 egg with 15 ml/1 level tablespoon skimmed milk. Meanwhile, grill 2 rashers streaky bacon. Serve the bacon and egg with 1 × 25 g/1 oz slice wholemeal toast topped with 5 ml/1 level teaspoon low-fat spread.

BELOW: Sausages and baked beans.

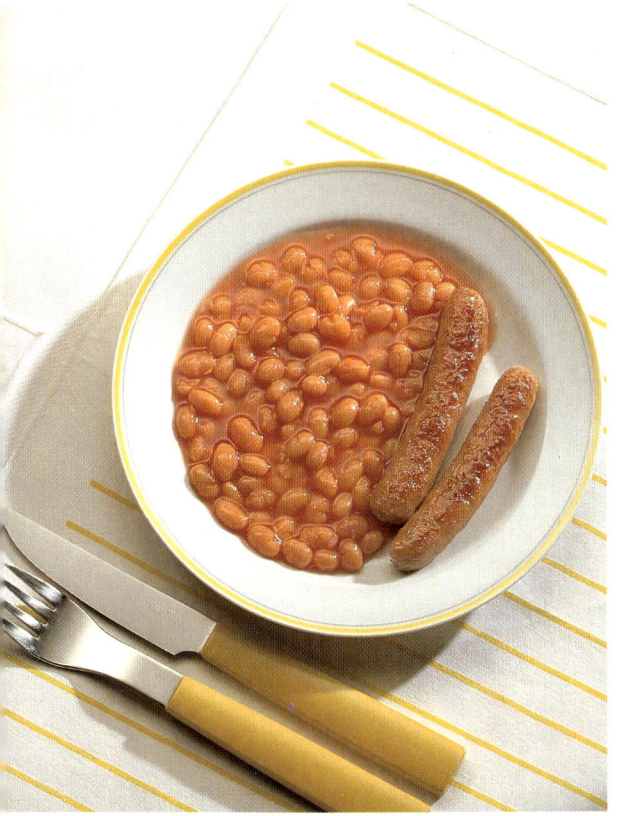

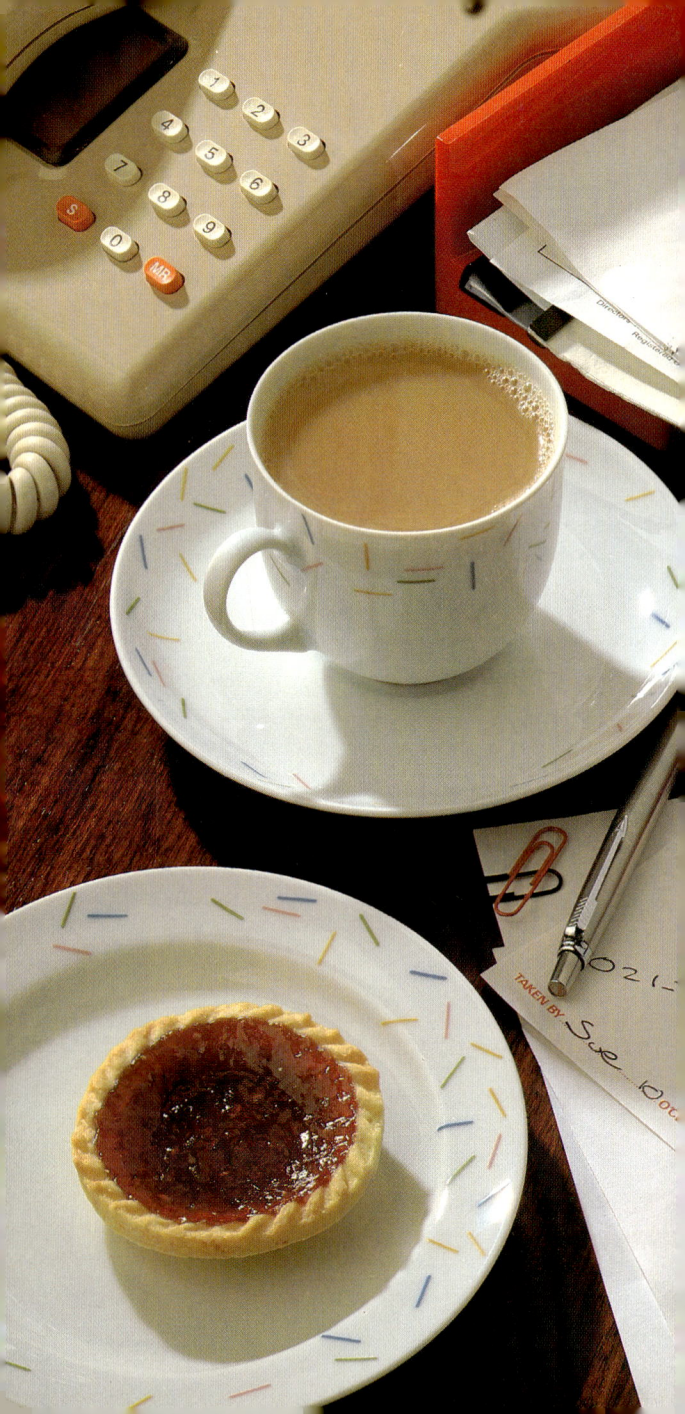

THE TEA TROLLEY

A snack from the office tea trolley or canteen can be very calorie costly. If you order a roll or piece of cake more out of habit than hunger, cutting out these snacks is an easy way to cut calories. However, if having nothing with your mid-morning coffee or afternoon tea sets you longing for bacon rolls and cream doughnuts, your best plan is to allow for this indulgence in your daily calories. One way to avoid temptation is to get your secretary to divert the tea trolley before it reaches your office door!

Savoury snacks

Bacon roll	280
Cheese and pickle roll	300
Corned beef roll	300
Crisps, per small packet, any flavour	150
Ham roll	240
Sausage roll (with bread roll)	325
Sausage roll (pastry)	400
Tuna and tomato roll	290

Biscuits

Per average biscuit:

Chocolate Chip Cookie	60
Digestive, large	70
Digestive, medium	55
Digestive, small	45
Fig Roll	65
Garibaldi, per finger	30
Ginger Nut	40
Ginger Snap	35
Jaffa Cake	50
Lincoln	40
Malted Milk	40
Marie	30
Morning Coffee	25
Nice	45
Rich Osborne	35
Rich Tea Finger	25

Rich Tea Round	45
Sponge Finger	20
Thin Arrowroot	30

Cakes

Homemade and bakery cakes
Per average slice or small cake:

Butterfly cake	200
Chelsea bun	255
Cherry cake	250
Chocolate cake, filled with butter icing and topped with chocolate glacé icing	525
Christmas cake or wedding cake, with marzipan and royal icing	350
Currant bun	150
Eccles cake	200
Flapjack	300
Fruit cake	300
Jam tart	110
Madeira cake	335
Mince pie	185
Scone, plain	210
Sponge sandwich, jam-filled, whisked fatless method	130
Victoria sandwich, jam-filled	260

Fresh cream cakes
Per average cake:

Chocolate éclair	275
Cream doughnut	260
Cream slice, with puff pastry and glacé icing	420
Meringue	195
Strawberry tart	200

Individual packeted cakes

Almond slice	135
Apple and blackcurrant pie	180
Apple pie	200
Blackcurrant sundae	200
Cherry cake slice	200
Chocolate-covered mini roll	120
Cup cake	130
Eccles cake	160

Fondant fancy	110
French fancy	110
Fruit cake slice	200
Jam tart	120
Junior chocolate roll	120
Mince pie	195
Redcurrant and raspberry pie	190
Redcurrant and raspberry tart	270
Viennese fancy	130
Viennese split	85

Cakes and biscuits

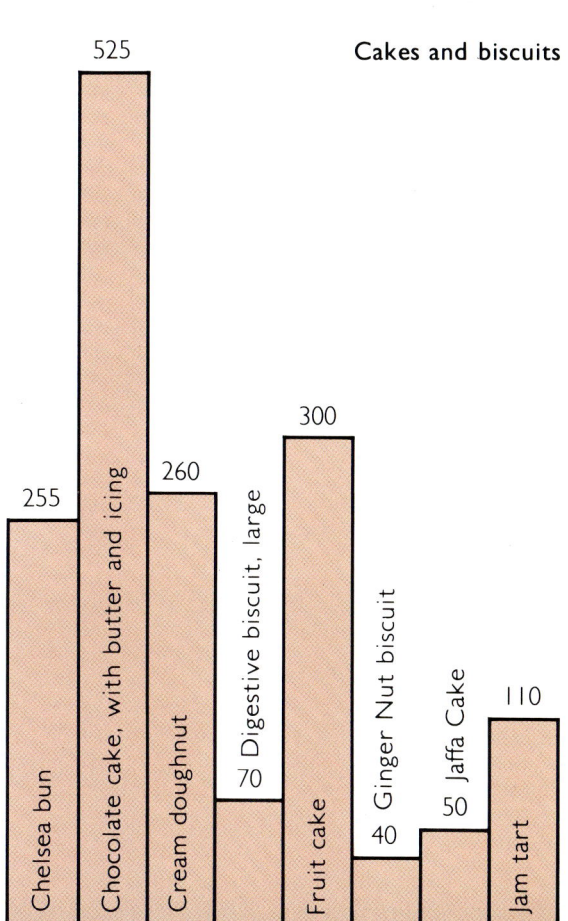

Chelsea bun — 255
Chocolate cake, with butter and icing — 525
Cream doughnut — 260
Digestive biscuit, large — 70
Fruit cake — 300
Ginger Nut biscuit — 40
Jaffa Cake — 50
Jam tart — 110

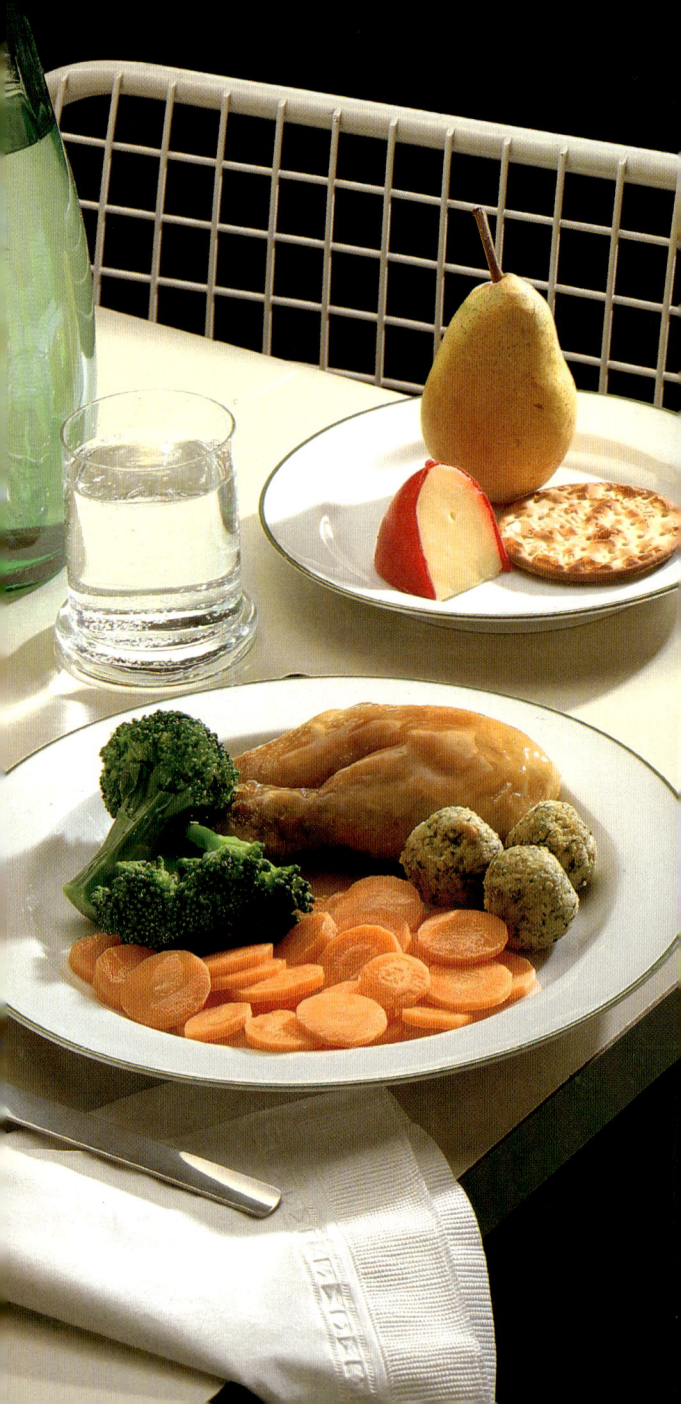

CANTEEN MEALS

The food that is served in work canteens or staff restaurants will vary according to the number catered for, workers' preferences and the whims of the catering manager. Some catering managers are very concerned with healthy eating and will provide low-fat, low-calorie meals, while other caterers may serve up more traditional fare.

It makes sense to approach your catering manager and ask him/her to put certain items on the regular menu. If this is practicable, most managers will be only too happy to oblige. In this chapter we list the most popular canteen dishes with their approximate calorie values.

Calorie cutters

- ★ Always cut off all visible fat from meat and leave it on the side of your plate.
- ★ Do not eat the skin from chicken, duck or turkey.
- ★ Say no to gravy and ask whoever serves you not to spoon buttery sauces over your meat or fish.

Breakfasts

Some canteens serve breakfast all morning, so if you prefer to miss breakfast at home and have a late morning brunch instead, choose from this list. But it's unlikely you'll be able to afford the 'full works' – fruit juice, a fry-up, toast, butter and marmalade can cost you over 900 Calories.

Fruit juices
Per 200 ml/7 fl oz glass:

Apple, unsweetened	70
Grapefruit, sweetened	75
Grapefruit, unsweetened	65
Orange, sweetened	100
Orange, unsweetened	75

Cereals

These are normally served in individual boxes. Allow 75 Calories for whole milk. If skimmed milk is available, allow 40 Calories. If you add sugar, allow 35 Calories per 10 ml/1 rounded teaspoon.

All Bran	105
Bran Flakes	85
Cornflakes	60
Muesli	150
Rice Krispies	75
Special K	60
Weetabix, 1 biscuit	65

Cooked breakfast items

Per average portion:

Bacon, 2 back rashers	160

Canteen breakfasts

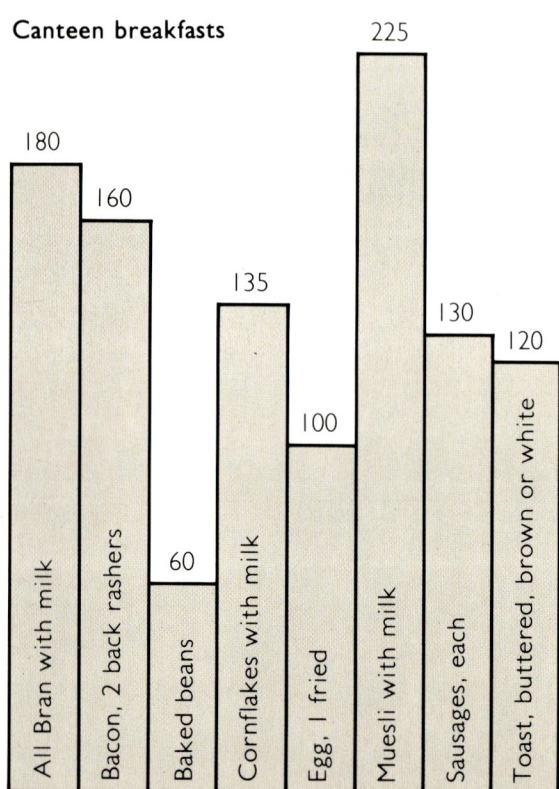

All Bran with milk	180
Bacon, 2 back rashers	160
Baked beans	60
Cornflakes with milk	135
Egg, 1 fried	100
Muesli with milk	225
Sausages, each	130
Toast, buttered, brown or white	120

Baked beans	60
Black pudding	170
Egg, 1 fried	100
Egg, 1 poached	80
Fried bread, 1 whole slice	180
Mushrooms, poached	10
Sausages, each	130
Sautéed potatoes	160
Tomatoes, each	10

Bread and toast

For butter and margarine, see the list of little extras. Toast is normally served ready buttered but most canteens will supply unbuttered toast if you ask.

Croissant	280
Crusty roll	145
Toast, brown, buttered, per slice	120
Toast, brown, unbuttered, per slice	75
Toast, white, buttered, per slice	120
Toast, white, unbuttered, per slice	75
Toast, wholemeal, buttered, per slice	115
Toast, wholemeal, unbuttered, per slice	70

Soups

Most canteens serve soups every day and usually make them from dehydrated mixes. Made-up dried soups nearly always work out lower in calories than canned or homemade soups. Eaten with just a crusty roll (145 Calories) or a slice of bread (75 Calories), they make a satisfying meal.

Per average portion:

Asparagus	110
Chicken noodle	75
French onion	60
Lentil	100
Minestrone	85
Oxtail	85
Pea	80
Scotch broth	70
Spring vegetable	50
Tomato	110
Vegetable and beef	90

Main courses

The following are some of the most popular main courses served in canteens. The calories for each meal will vary slightly from canteen to canteen, but the differences are not likely to be as great as with restaurant meals. The calories below are for the main dish only. For vegetables see the list on page 40. Calories for salads include the main item (e.g. cheese or ham) and a selection of the following vegetables: lettuce, cucumber, celery, carrot, tomato, cress. They do not include any salads mixed with dressing, such as coleslaw. If you wish to add dressing, salad cream or mayonnaise to your salad, see the list of little extras. With all meats, discard all visible fat before eating.

Under 150 Calories
Beef salad (1 slice beef)
Cottage cheese salad
Egg salad
Grilled fish
Ham salad (2 slices ham)
Pilchard salad
Prawn salad (without seafood sauce)

150 to 200 Calories
Corned beef salad (1 slice corned beef)
Grilled trout
Pork salad
Roast lamb with mint sauce and gravy
Salami salad

200 to 250 Calories
Cannelloni
Gammon and pineapple
Lamb chop
Lasagne
Luncheon meat salad
Roast chicken with stuffing and gravy
Roast pork, apple sauce, stuffing and gravy
Smoked mackerel salad
Tuna salad

250 to 300 Calories
Chicken salad (chicken without skin)
Hamburger (small) in bun with relish or tomato
　　ketchup
Mushroom omelette
Plain omelette
Pork chop
Roast beef, Yorkshire pudding and gravy
Sausages (2)
Steak, medium or well-grilled

300 to 350 Calories
Bacon omelette
Cheeseburger (small) in bun
Egg mayonnaise salad
Fish, fried in batter
Ham omelette
Liver and bacon
Steak, grilled rare

350 to 400 Calories
Beef and mushroom pie (with pastry top only)
Cheese omelette
Cheese salad
Chicken pie (with pastry top only)
Scampi with Tartare sauce
Scotch egg salad
Shepherd's pie
Steak and kidney pie (with pastry top only)

400 to 450 Calories
Beef and mushroom or beef and onion pie
　　(individual)
Cauliflower cheese
Chicken pie (individual)
Chicken salad (including skin)
Cornish pasty
Hamburger (quarterpounder) with bun and
　　relish or tomato ketchup
Pork and egg pie (slice from long pie)
Steak and kidney pie (individual)

450 to 500 Calories

Cheeseburger (quarterpounder) with bun and
  relish or tomato ketchup
Quiche or egg and bacon flan
Toasted steak sandwich

Main courses

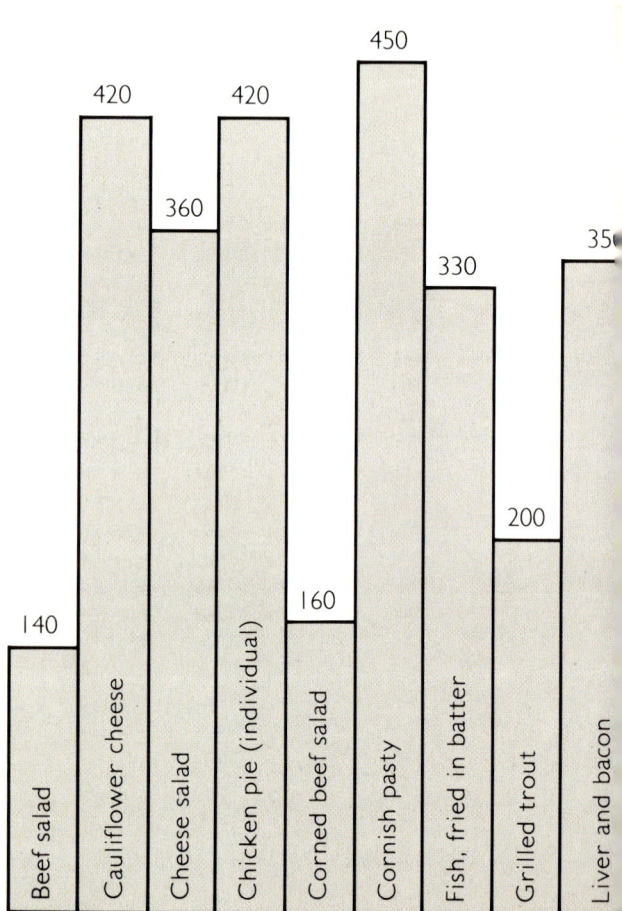

Over 500 Calories
Beef stew and dumplings
Macaroni cheese
Meat curry and rice
Pork pie (individual) and salad
Spaghetti Bolognese
Steak and kidney pudding

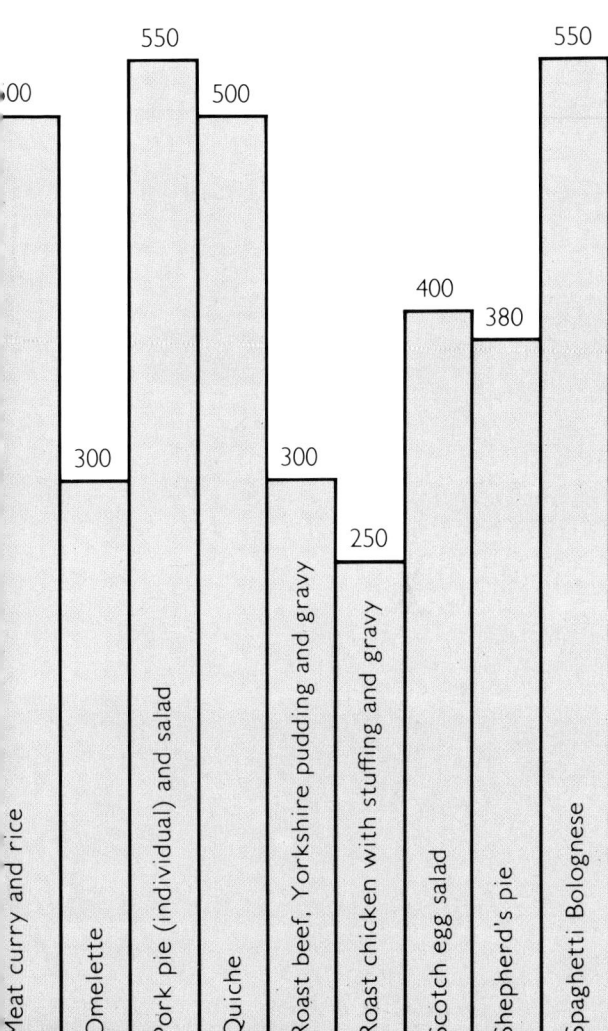

Meat curry and rice	00	
Omelette	300	
Pork pie (individual) and salad	550	
Quiche	500	
Roast beef, Yorkshire pudding and gravy	300	
Roast chicken with stuffing and gravy	250	
Scotch egg salad	400	
Shepherd's pie	380	
Spaghetti Bolognese	550	

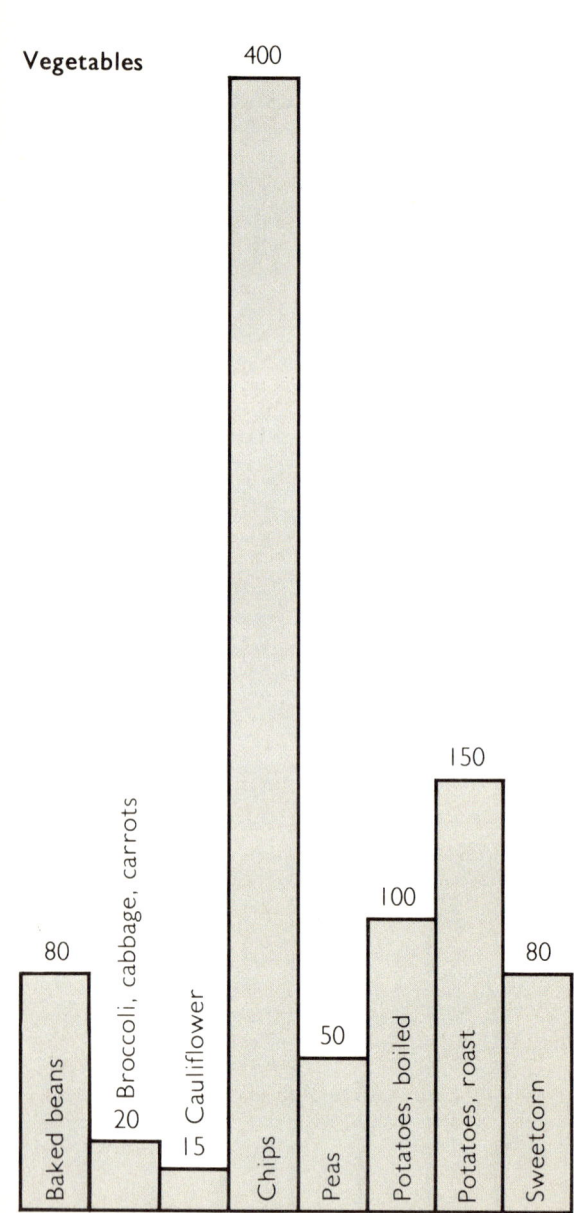

Vegetables

Baked beans 80
Broccoli, cabbage, carrots 20
Cauliflower 15
Chips 400
Peas 50
Potatoes, boiled 100
Potatoes, roast 150
Sweetcorn 80

Vegetables

Scarcely any canteens add butter to their vegetables, so they are far lower in calories and fat than in restaurants. The only vegetables to avoid altogether are those cooked in fat – chips and roast potatoes, for instance – or any that are served in sauce, such as cauliflower in cheese sauce.

Per average portion:

Baked beans	80
Broad beans	40
Broccoli	20
Brussels sprouts	20
Cabbage	20
Carrots	20
Cauliflower	15
Cauliflower in cheese sauce	250
Chips	400
Green beans	20
Mixed vegetables	50
Peas	50
Potatoes, boiled	100
Potatoes, creamed	130
Potatoes, roast	150
Potatoes, sautéed	200
Sweetcorn	80

Puddings and desserts

Top of the popularity charts for canteen puds are diet-destroying, high-calorie desserts, such as rhubarb crumble and custard and treacle tart. But nearly all canteens sell fresh fruit or ice cream and these provide the best way to finish off a meal when you are on a diet. The calories below do not include custard, cream or ice cream toppings unless stated.

Less than 100 Calories
Fresh fruit (1 piece)
Ice cream (1 scoop)

100 to 150 Calories
Choc ice
Custard
Fresh fruit salad
Fruit in jelly
Fruit yogurt

150 to 200 Calories
Crême caramel
Rice pudding
Semolina pudding
Tapioca pudding

200 to 250 Calories
Bread and butter pudding
Mousse, any flavour
Stewed fruit and custard
Trifle

250 to 300 Calories
Fruit flan
Ice cream with canned fruit
Ice cream with sauce and nuts

300 to 350 Calories
Apple strudel
Fruit pie (pastry on top only)

350 to 400 Calories
Chocolate gâteau with fruit and cream
Lemon meringue pie
Sponge gâteau with fruit and cream

Over 400 Calories
Bread pudding
Cheesecake
Fruit crumble
Fruit pie (pastry top and bottom)
Jam roly poly
Spotted Dick
Treacle tart

Cheese and biscuits

Canteen cheeses usually come in packets or ready-weighed portions.

Cheese
Per individual portion:

Austrian smoked	140
Babybel	75
Bel Paese	85
Camembert	125
Cheddar	180
Cheshire	165
Danish blue	90
Double Gloucester	160
Edam	130
Lancashire	165
Leicester	160
Stilton	195

Biscuits

Cream cracker	35
Digestive biscuit	55
Ryvita	25
Water biscuit	30

Sauces and extras

Most canteens serve sauces, butters and preserves in individual catering packs. The sizes and calories of these only vary slightly from brand to brand.

Sauces and pickles
Per individual pack:

Brown sauce, tub pack	30
Horseradish sauce	10
Mustard, squeeze pack	10
Piccalilli, tub pack	10
Salad cream, tub pack	70
Sweet pickle, tub pack	15
Tartare sauce, squeeze pack	30
Tartare sauce, tub pack	55
Thousand Island dressing, squeeze pack	50
Tomato ketchup, squeeze pack	15
Tomato ketchup, tub pack	20

Other salad dressings

It is unlikely that you will find a canteen that supplies a low-calorie dressing, but they may well have bowls of mayonnaise or dressing from which you can help yourself. Mayonnaise and French dressing are both extremely high in calories so you can't afford carelessly to tip a dollop onto your salad. Here is what a *carefully* measured amount would cost.

Per 15 ml/1 level tablespoon:

French dressing	75
Mayonnaise	120
Salad cream	50

Butter

Per individual pack:

All brands	80

Honey, jam and marmalade

Per individual pack:

Honey, clear	60
Honey, set	70
Jam	65
Marmalade	65

Milk and milk substitutes

Per individual pack:

Coffee creamer	20
Half cream	20
Milk	10
Single cream	30
Skimmed milk powder	10

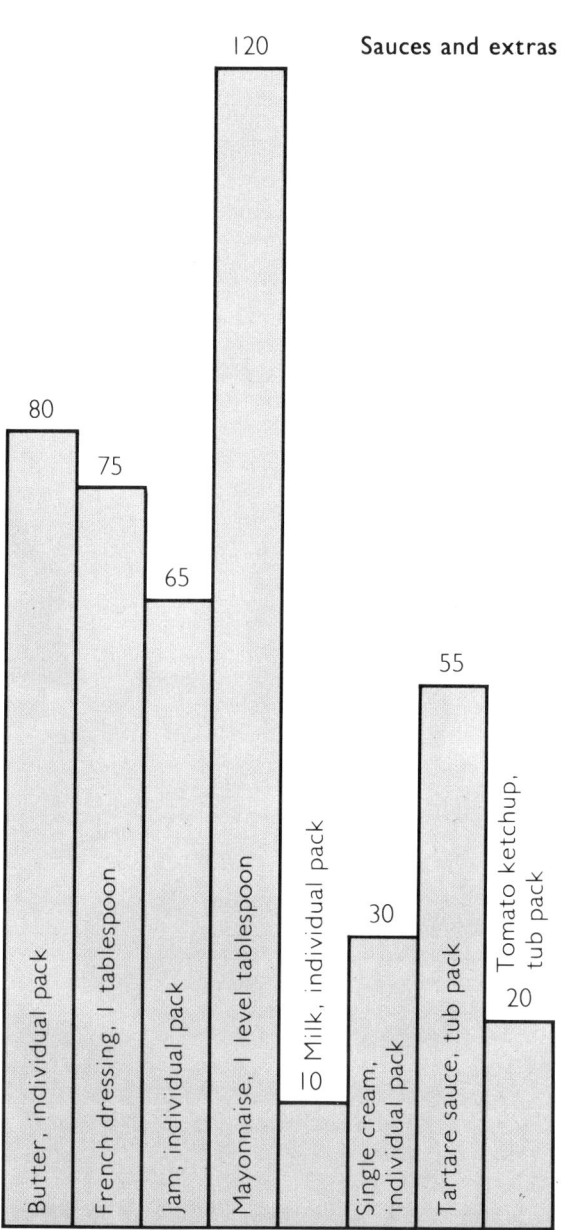

Sauces and extras

120 — Mayonnaise, 1 level tablespoon
80 — Butter, individual pack
75 — French dressing, 1 tablespoon
65 — Jam, individual pack
55 — Tartare sauce, tub pack
30 — Single cream, individual pack
20 — Tomato ketchup, tub pack
10 — Milk, individual pack

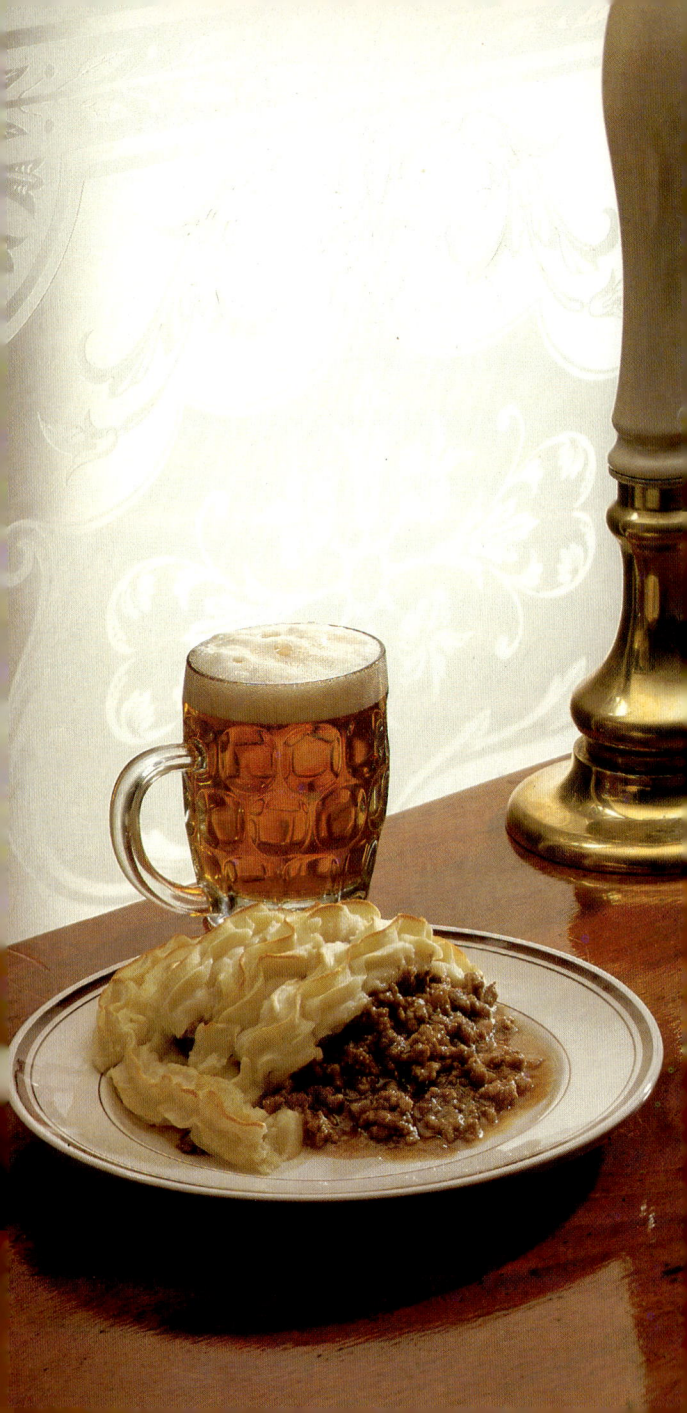

PUB AND WINE BAR LUNCHES

Pubs and wine bars are a law unto themselves when it comes to serving food. Some pubs and wine bars specialize in homemade pies and casseroles, while other establishments may rely on ready-made meals from catering suppliers.

Below we give a very approximate guide to what a pub or wine bar meal will cost. Portions and ingredients used vary so enormously that one pub's cannelloni could easily be 100 Calories more than its neighbour's. To be on the safe side, count the highest calories in each group. See page 79 on calories for alcoholic drinks.

Calorie cutters

* An individual foil-wrapped butter pat costs about 80 Calories, and you'll make a worthwhile saving if you hand this back to the barman. Spread your French bread with pickle instead of butter when you eat a ploughman's lunch.
* Try a spritzer for a change – $\frac{1}{2}$ wine and $\frac{1}{2}$ soda or sparkling mineral water. It's great on a hot day and you'll get twice the quantity for the same calories as a glass of wine.
* If there is a help-yourself salad bar where you eat, choose a green salad without dressing and avoid anything covered in mayonnaise or oil.

---

200 to 300 Calories
Hamburger (small) in bun with relish or tomato ketchup

Minestrone or thick vegetable soup with roll (no butter)

Pizza (small), approximately 13 cm/5 inches in diameter

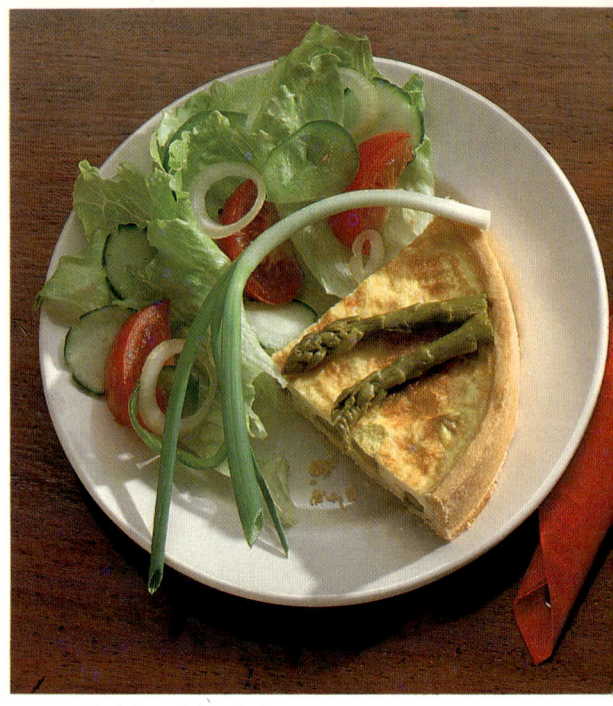

ABOVE: *Quiche with salad.*

300 to 400 Calories

Baked potato with cheese (no butter)
Cheeseburger (small) in bun with relish or
  tomato ketchup
Chilli con carne
Minestrone or thick vegetable soup with roll
  and butter
Shepherd's pie with brown sauce or tomato
  ketchup
Toasted cheese and ham sandwich
Toasted cheese sandwich
Tomato soup and roll (no butter)

400 to 500 Calories

Cannelloni
Pizza (approximately 18 cm/7 inches in diameter)
Toasted steak sandwich
Tomato soup with roll and butter

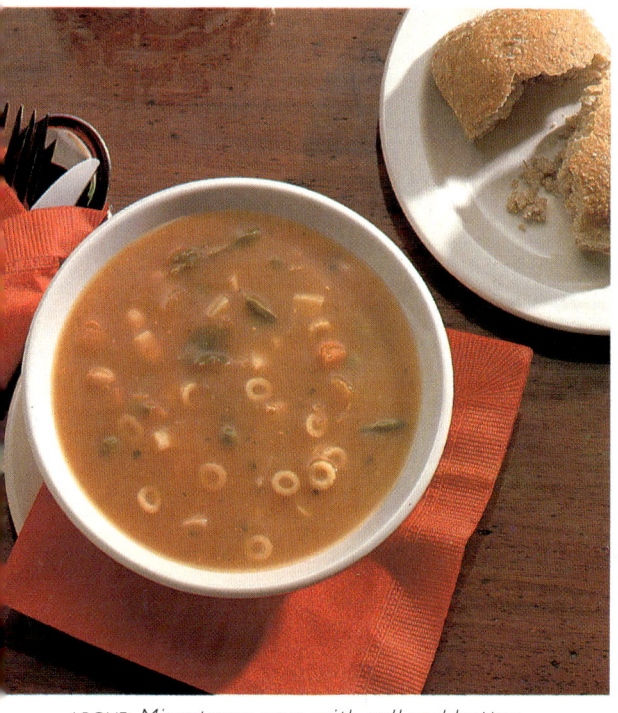
ABOVE: Minestrone soup with roll and butter.

500 to 600 Calories
Brie with French bread (no butter)
Lasagne
Moussaka
Pork pie and salad (no dressing)
Quarterpounder hamburger with relish or
  tomato ketchup
Quiche with salad (no dressing)
Sausage (1) with French bread and pickle (no
  butter)

600 to 700 Calories
Brie with French bread, salad garnish and butter
Cheeseburger, quarterpounder, with relish or
  tomato ketchup
Ploughman's, without butter
Sausages (2) with French bread and pickle (no
  butter)

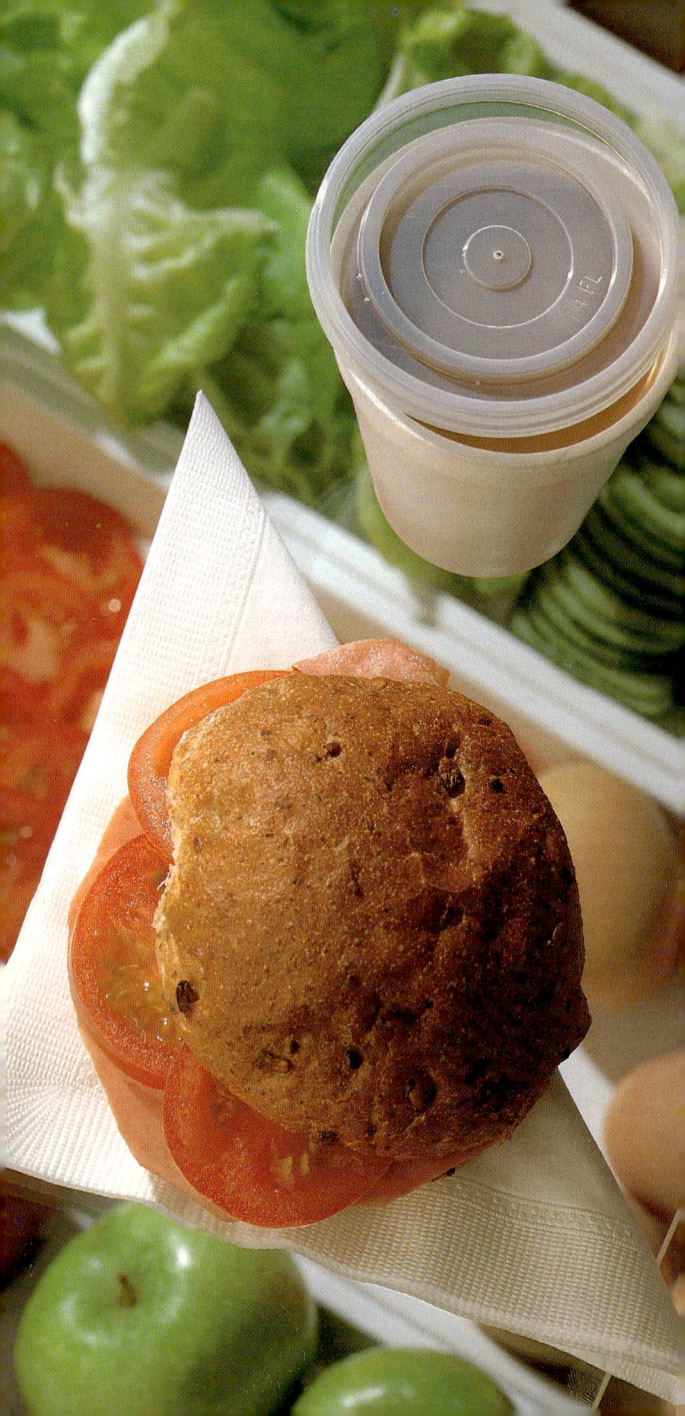

BOUGHT ROLLS AND SANDWICHES

If you buy rolls or sandwiches for lunch from a local café or sandwich bar, here is approximately what they will cost you. Most places will use 2 lightly buttered slices of bread for sandwiches and a medium-size roll, but fillings do vary. For instance, one place may fill a prawn sandwich with a generous 25 g/1 oz prawns mixed with a little mayonnaise, whereas another bar may be mean with the prawns and generous with the mayonnaise. Usually, though, the more expensive the roll or sandwich, the bigger chunk it is likely to take out of your calorie allowance.

Calorie cutters

* If you buy from a sandwich bar that makes up rolls and sandwiches while you wait, ask them not to butter the bread. This will save you about 100 Calories for a sandwich and 50 Calories for a roll.
* If you have access to hot water at lunchtime, keep some low-calorie sachet soups in your office drawer and drink one of these with your roll or sandwich. You'll find it far more filling than drinking tea or coffee and it will only cost you about 40 Calories.
* If you buy a meat sandwich or roll, open it up and discard any visible fat before you eat.
* A medium-size crusty roll will weigh about 45 g/1¾ oz. Some large soft wholemeal rolls can weigh 150 g/5 oz and add 300 Calories to your bought-butty total. If you are in doubt, borrow a postal scale and weigh the roll.

Rolls

Calories allow for a medium-size crusty round roll.
It does not matter whether you choose brown or
white. For a wholemeal roll you can knock off 20
Calories.

Bacon	280
Beef and mustard	270
Cheese	290
Cheese and pickle	300
Cheese and tomato	300
Corned beef and pickle	300
Cottage cheese and pickle	260
Cream cheese and cucumber	330
Egg mayonnaise	320
Ham	240
Ham and tomato	250
Liver sausage	290
Prawn mayonnaise	300
Salad	270
Salmon and cucumber	270
Tuna	290

Sandwiches

Each sandwich is calculated on 2 slices of lightly
buttered bread.

Bacon	430
Beef and mustard	360
Cheese	400
Cheese and pickle	410
Cheese and tomato	400
Cream cheese and cucumber	400
Corned beef and pickle	350
Cottage cheese and pickle	340
Egg mayonnaise	450
Ham	320
Ham and tomato	330
Liver sausage	450
Prawn mayonnaise	420
Salad	280
Salmon and cucumber	360
Tuna	400

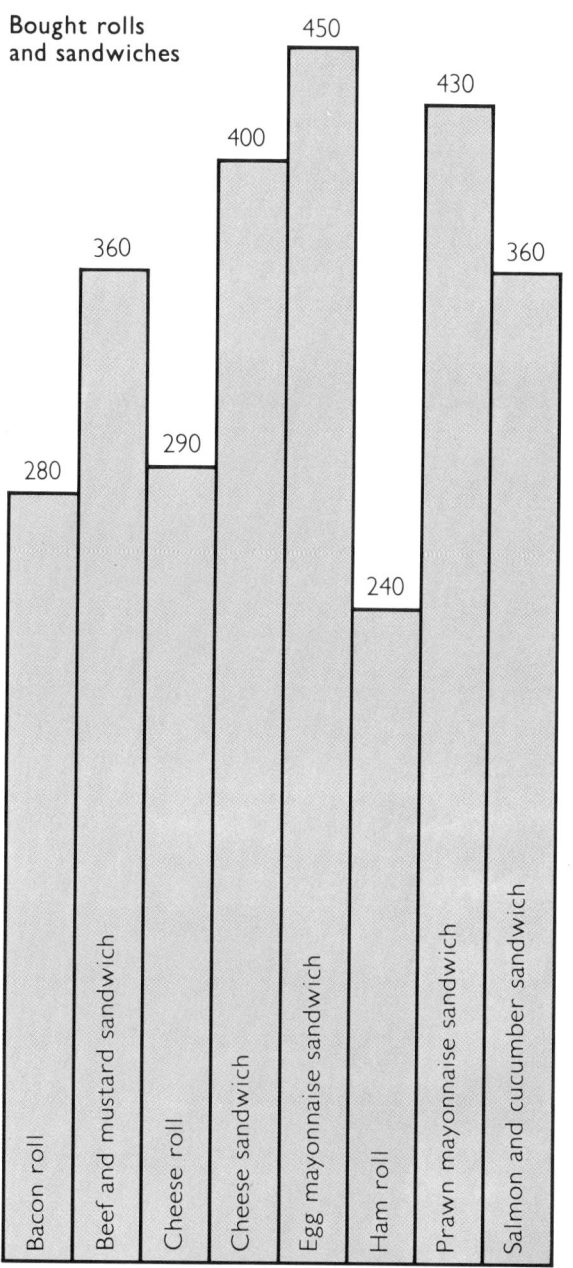

Bought rolls and sandwiches

- 280 Bacon roll
- 360 Beef and mustard sandwich
- 290 Cheese roll
- 400 Cheese sandwich
- 450 Egg mayonnaise sandwich
- 240 Ham roll
- 430 Prawn mayonnaise sandwich
- 360 Salmon and cucumber sandwich

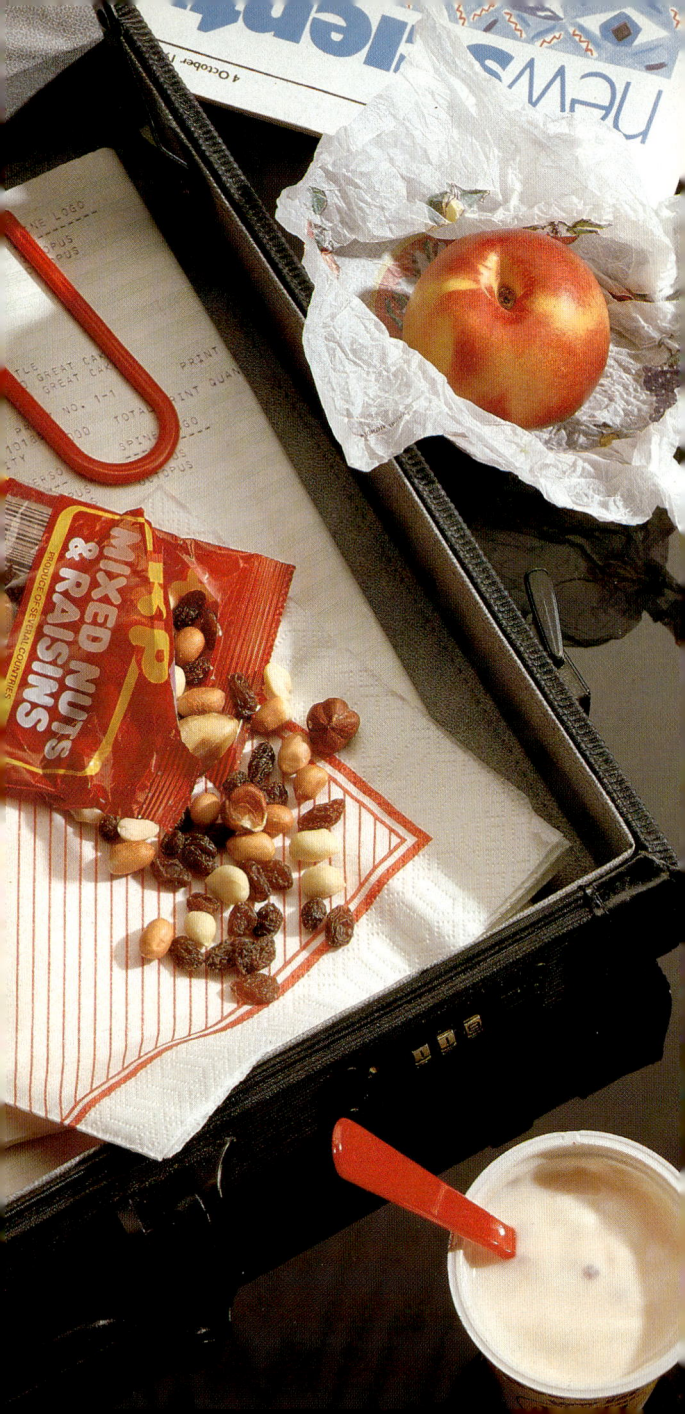

DESK-BOUND LUNCHES

You'll get the best value for your calories if you take a packed lunch to the office. Unlike businesswomen, many men seem a little shy when it comes to munching a home-packed salad at their desks, and we have therefore included only a few salads and concentrated more on sandwich meals and made them all total about 350 Calories for easy counting. On a nice day you could eat your packed lunch in a nearby park – remember that walking will burn up extra calories (it will make you feel more mentally refreshed, too).

Calorie cutters

★ Have curd or low-fat skimmed milk soft cheese instead of cream cheese and save 70 to 100 Calories per 25 g/1 oz.
★ Take care that you choose tuna in brine for your homemade sandwiches rather than tuna in oil. When canned in brine, tuna is just 30 Calories per drained 25 g/1 oz. Canned in oil, it doubles its calories even if you drain the oil away. Mash the oil with the tuna and the calories soar up to over 80 per 25 g/1 oz.

Bought butties

All these lunches-for-one are based on a standard size sandwich or a plain, round crusty bread roll, bought ready-filled from a shop, sandwich bar or canteen.

Salad roll plus yogurt
350 Calories

Start with 1 salad roll. To follow, have 1 × 150 g/ 5 oz carton low-fat fruit yogurt, any flavour.

Cheese and tomato roll plus fruit
350 Calories

Start with 1 cheese and tomato roll. To follow, have 1 medium apple or 1 small banana.

Cottage cheese and pickle roll plus fruit
350 Calories

Start with 1 cottage cheese and pickle roll. To follow, have 1 large banana or 2 medium apples.

Ham and tomato roll plus fruit
350 Calories

Start with 1 ham and tomato roll. To follow, have 175 g/6 oz grapes or 225 g/8 oz fresh cherries.

Salmon and cucumber roll plus fruit
350 Calories

Start with 1 salmon and cucumber roll. To follow, have 1 large peach or 1 large orange.

Beef sandwich
350 Calories

Have 1 beef sandwich, with mustard if liked.

Corned beef and pickle sandwich
350 Calories

Have 1 corned beef and pickle sandwich.

Packed lunches to take to work

Sardine and olive sandwich plus fruit
350 Calories

Mash 2 canned sardines in tomato sauce. Stir in 2 olives, sliced. Place between 2 × 40g/1½oz slices wholemeal bread. Follow with 125 g/4 oz grapes.

Tuna and cucumber sandwich plus fruit
350 Calories

Drain and mash 1 × 100 g/3½ oz can tuna in brine.
Mix with 15 ml/1 tablespoon low-calorie seafood
sauce or low-calorie salad dressing. Use with a few
slices of cucumber as a filling for 2 × 40 g/1½ oz slices
wholemeal bread. To follow, have 1 medium pear
or apple.

Stilton and celery roll plus fruit
350 Calories

Grate 25 g/1 oz Blue Stilton cheese. Chop a small
piece of celery. Mix the cheese and celery with
25 g/1 oz cottage cheese with chives and 5 ml/1
teaspoon low-calorie salad dressing. Use as a filling
for 1 crusty brown or white bread roll. To follow,
have 1 medium apple or pear.

─────── Calorie cutters ───────

★ Is cheese your favourite filling? Choose
Edam instead of Cheddar and the calories
come down from 120 to 90 per 25 g/1 oz.
Or get to know the new, reduced-fat
cheeses – Tendale Cheddar-type cheese is
just 70 Calories per 25 g/1 oz.

Cheese and chutney roll plus fruit
350 Calories

Split 1 crusty brown or white bread roll and spread
with 15 ml/1 level tablespoon mango chutney. Fill
with 25 g/1 oz grated Lancashire or Leicestershire
cheese. To follow, have 1 medium apple or orange.

Sausage and potato roll plus fruit
350 Calories

Grill 1 pork chipolata sausage well. When cool,
slice thinly. Dice 40 g/1½ oz cooked potato, and
chop 1 small spring onion or a few chives. Mix the
vegetables with 15 ml/1 level tablespoon low-
calorie salad dressing. Use, with the sausage, as a
filling for 1 crusty brown or white bread roll. To
follow, have 1 medium banana or 1 large orange.

Cottage cheese and peanut sandwich plus fruit
350 Calories

Roughly chop 15 ml/1 level tablespoon roasted or dry-roasted peanuts. Mix with 50 g/2 oz natural cottage cheese and 2.5 ml/½ level teaspoon Marmite. Use as a filling between 2 × 40 g/1½ oz slices wholemeal bread. To follow, have 1 medium apple or banana.

Cheese spread, tomato and pickle sandwiches
350 Calories

Make 2 sandwiches using 4 × 25 g/1 oz slices wholemeal bread, 25 g/1 oz cheese spread, 1 medium sliced tomato and 20 ml/4 level teaspoons sweet pickle.

Egg and cress sandwich plus fruit
350 Calories

Hard-boil 1 size 3 egg. When cool, chop the egg finely and mix with 15 ml/1 level tablespoon low-calorie salad dressing. Stir in some cress and use the mixture to fill 2 × 40 g/1½ oz slices wholemeal bread. To follow, have 125 g/4 oz grapes.

Beef sandwich plus fruit
350 Calories

Cut off and discard all visible fat from 50 g/2 oz thinly sliced roast topside of beef. Combine 15 ml/1 level tablespoon low-fat spread with 2.5–5 ml/½–1 level teaspoon prepared mustard or creamed horseradish. Spread on 2 × 40 g/1½ oz slices wholemeal bread, and make a sandwich with the beef. To follow, have 1 medium peach or pear.

Ham and tomato sandwich plus fruit
350 Calories

Discard all visible fat from 40 g/1½ oz lean cooked ham. Spread 2 × 40 g/1½ oz slices wholemeal bread with 15 ml/1 level tablespoon low-fat spread and fill with the ham, topped with 1 sliced tomato. To follow, have 1 medium apple or 1 small banana.

Chicken and sweetcorn sandwich plus fruit
350 Calories

Chop 50 g/2 oz skinless cooked chicken; mix with 25 g/1 oz drained canned or cooked sweetcorn and 15 ml/1 level tablespoon low-calorie salad dressing. Use as a filling between 2 × 40 g/1½ oz slices wholemeal bread. To follow, have 1 medium peach or pear.

Supermarket diet savers

If you forget to take lunch to work, you can buy these items from a supermarket.

Camembert and bread roll plus fruit
350 Calories

Have 1 × 40 g/1½ oz individual wedge of Camembert cheese and 1 brown or white crusty bread roll. To follow, have 125 g/4 oz grapes or 1 medium banana.

Nuts and raisins plus yogurt and fruit
350 Calories

Have 1 × 40 g/1½ oz packet nuts and raisins plus 1 × 150 g/5 oz carton low-fat fruit yogurt. To follow, have 1 mandarin, satsuma, tangerine or peach.

Cottage cheese plus crisps and fruit
350 Calories

Have 1 × 113 g/4 oz carton cottage cheese with

Calorie cutter

* Is eating your automatic response to stress? Take a walk instead or relax with a low-calorie drink.

Cheddar and onion plus 1 × 25 g/1 oz packet potato crisps, any flavour. To follow, have 150 g/5 oz fresh cherries or 125 g/4 oz grapes.

Cottage cheese with prawns and crispbreads plus fruit
350 Calories

Have 1 × 170 g/6 oz carton cottage cheese with prawns with 3 Ryvita or high fibre crispbreads. To follow, have 1 large apple or orange.

Soup and roll plus yogurt
350 Calories

Make up 1 sachet soup-in-a-cup. Choose from beef and onion, beef and tomato, golden vegetable, oxtail, and spring vegetable flavours. Serve with 1 wholemeal bread roll. To follow, have 1 × 150 g/ 5 oz carton low-fat fruit yogurt, any flavour.

Carton salads

Many men seem to feel that taking a carton of salad to work does not fit in with their image. If you can overcome this prejudice, you will find that the following salads are substantial and delicious. Pack them in a plastic container and take a spoon to work to eat them with. They are all easy to prepare and can be made the night before and stored in the refrigerator. All the salads serve 1.

Chicken and pasta salad
350 Calories

40 g/1½ oz wholewheat pasta rings or shapes
75 g/3 oz frozen peas
1 stick celery
¼ red pepper
50 g/2 oz cooked chicken or turkey
15 ml/1 level tablespoon low-fat natural yogurt
30 ml/2 level tablespoons low-calorie salad
  dressing
salt and pepper

Boil the pasta until just tender. Drain, rinse under cold water and drain again. Boil the peas for 5 minutes. Drain, rinse under cold water and drain again. Thinly slice the celery. Dice the pepper. Discard skin from the chicken or turkey and cut the flesh into bite-sized pieces. Add the yogurt and dressing, mix all ingredients together and season. Pack into a plastic container and refrigerate until needed.

Chicken, rice and raisin salad
350 Calories

40 g/1½ oz brown or white long-grain rice
50 g/2 oz cooked chicken, skinned and chopped
¼ red or green pepper, cored, seeded and diced
50 g/2 oz canned or cooked sweetcorn, drained
30 ml/2 level tablespoons raisins or sultanas
30 ml/2 tablespoons oil-free French dressing
salt and pepper

Cook the rice in plenty of boiling water until tender. Drain and leave to cool. Mix all ingredients and season lightly. Pack into a plastic container and refrigerate until needed.

Pasta and salmon salad
350 Calories

40 g/1½ oz white or wholewheat pasta shapes
50 g/2 oz frozen peas
¼ red or green pepper, cored, seeded and diced
75 g/3 oz canned salmon, drained and flaked
2 olives, sliced
15 ml/1 tablespoon oil-free French dressing
15 ml/1 level tablespoon low-calorie salad
  dressing
salt and pepper

Boil the pasta and peas separately until tender. Drain and leave to cool. Combine with remaining ingredients. Season lightly with salt and pepper. Pack into a plastic container and refrigerate until needed.

Red bean and tuna salad plus fruit
350 Calories

1 × 100 g/3½ oz can tuna in brine, drained and
   flaked
1 × 227 g/8 oz can red kidney beans, drained
1 stick celery, sliced
1 spring onion, sliced
1 tomato, sliced
15 ml/1 tablespoon oil-free French dressing
15 ml/1 level tablespoon tomato chutney
pepper
1 medium apple or pear

Mix all the ingredients except the fruit together.
Season with pepper. Pack into a plastic container
and refrigerate until needed. Pack fruit separately.

BELOW: Red bean and tuna salad plus fruit.

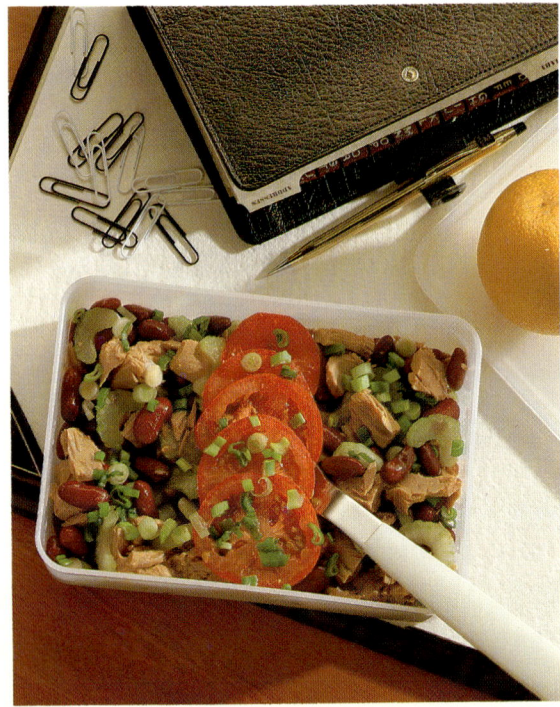

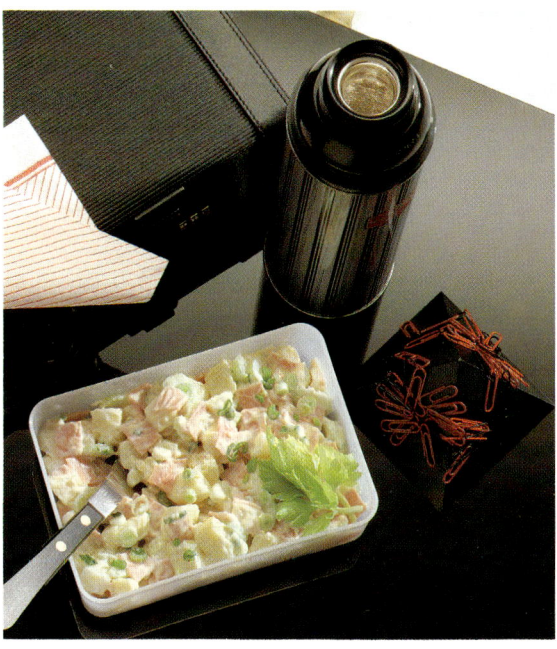

ABOVE: Potato and ham salad.

Potato and ham salad
350 Calories

225 g/8 oz potatoes, preferably new
50 g/2 oz lean cooked ham
30 ml/2 level tablespoons low-calorie salad
    dressing
15 ml/1 level tablespoon low-fat natural yogurt
salt and pepper
1 or 2 spring onions, chopped
1 stick celery, chopped

Cook the potatoes in boiling water, drain, cool and
dice. Remove all visible fat from the ham and dice.
Mix the salad dressing with the yogurt and season
with salt and pepper. Combine the potatoes, ham
and vegetables and stir in the mixed dressing. Pack
into a plastic container and refrigerate until
needed.

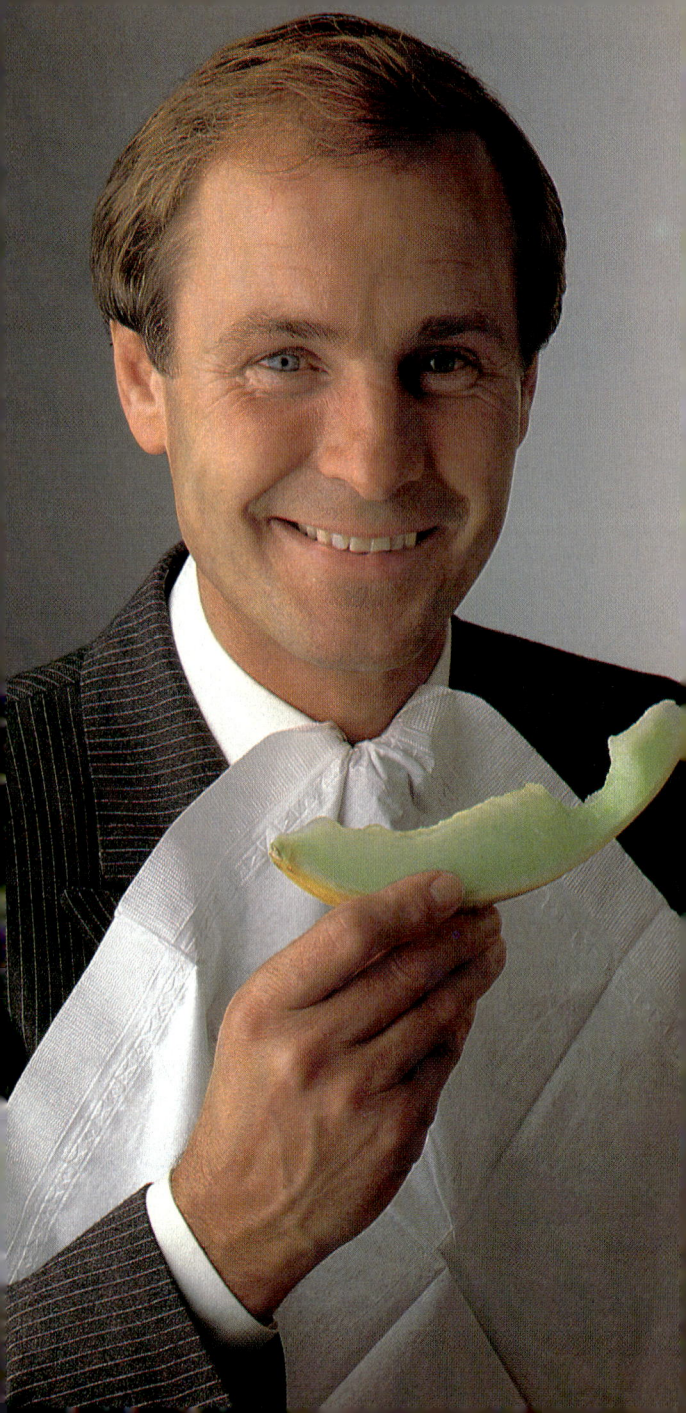

FRESH FRUIT

Fresh fruit makes a good low-calorie dessert or snack between meals. Here is a chart to show what an average piece or portion will cost you.

Apple, 1 medium	50
Apple, 1 large	80
Apricots, 225 g/8 oz	60
Banana, 1 small	50
Banana, 1 medium	80
Banana, 1 large	100
Cherries, 125 g/4 oz	50
Clementine, each	20
Dates, 4 medium	60
Figs, each	30
Grapes, 125 g/4 oz	70
Grapefruit, 1 whole medium	40
Kiwi fruit, 1 medium	30
Mandarin, 1 medium	20
Mango, 1 medium	100
Melon, cantaloupe, honeydew, 350 g/12 oz slice	50
Melon, Galia or Ogen, 1 medium $\frac{1}{2}$	50
Nectarine, 1 medium	50
Orange, 1 small	40
Orange, 1 medium	50
Orange, 1 large	80
Papaya, 1 medium	100
Passion fruit, 1 whole	5
Peach, 1 medium	40
Peach, 1 large	70
Pear, 1 medium	40
Pear, 1 large	80
Pineapple, 1 × 200 g/7 oz slice, weighed with skin and core	50
Pink grapefruit, 1 medium	30
Plums, 4 dessert	60
Pomegranate, 1 whole	65
Raspberries, 225 g/8 oz	60
Satsuma, 1 medium	20
Strawberries, 225 g/8 oz	60
Tangerine, 1 medium	20

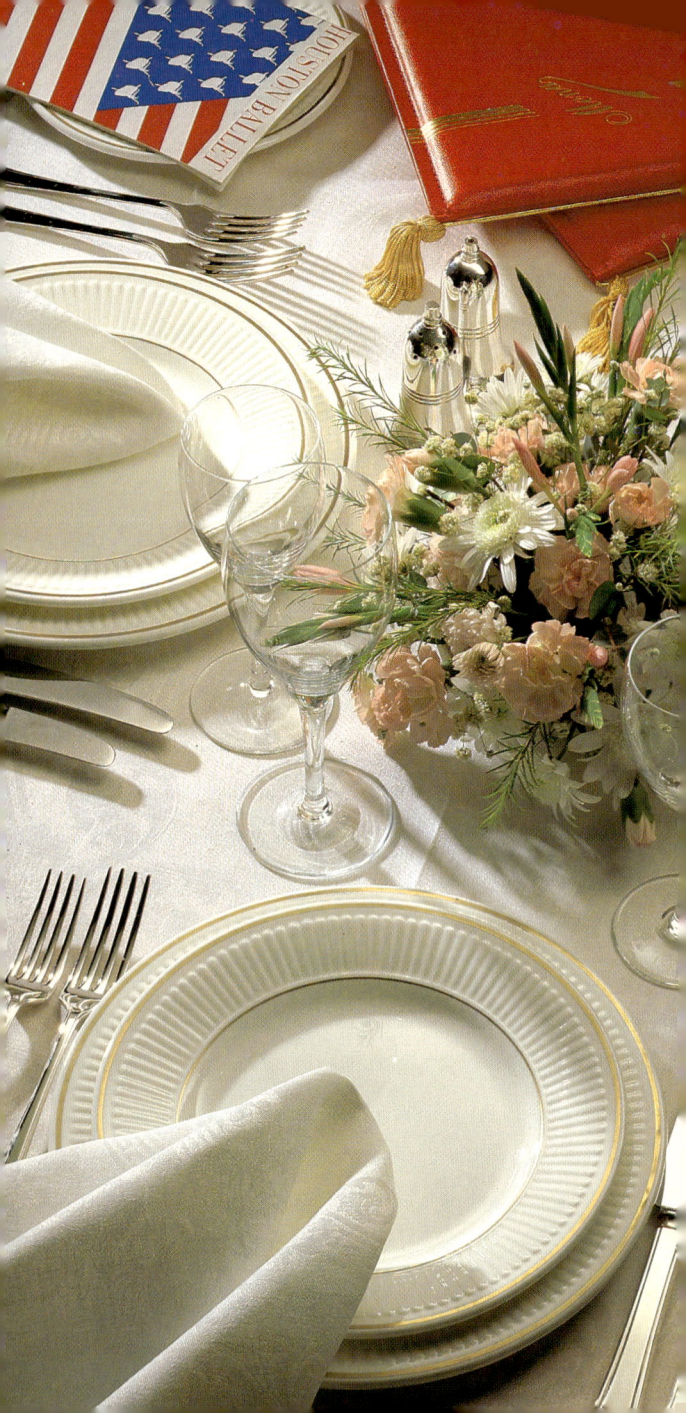

RESTAURANT MEALS

Recipes and portion sizes vary enormously from restaurant to restaurant, which makes it impossible for us to give accurate calorie counts for most dishes. However, this guide of approximate values will enable you to select a menu to fit into your diet.

Calories for the main course are for the dish with its sauce and garnish only. You will need to add on calories for salads or vegetables served with the dish from the list on pages 76–77.

Calorie cutter

★ Don't nibble rolls and butter as you wait for your meal unless you count the calorie cost. A crusty roll costs 145 Calories and a 15 g/$\frac{1}{2}$ oz portion of butter will add another 105 Calories.

Starters

Under 100 Calories
Consommé
Florida cocktail
Fruit juice
Grapefruit cocktail
Grapefruit, fresh $\frac{1}{2}$
Melon
Oysters with lemon (without brown bread and butter)
Smoked salmon (without brown bread and butter)
Tomato juice

100 to 200 Calories
Asparagus with butter
Corn on the cob without butter
Crab and sweetcorn soup
Crudités with dip

Lobster cocktail (without brown bread and
 butter)
Minestrone soup
Mushrooms à la Grecque
Parma ham with fresh figs
Parma ham with melon
Potted shrimps (without brown bread and
 butter)
Prawn cocktail (without brown bread and
 butter)
Prawn and tomato soup
Smoked eel (without brown bread and butter)
Smoked trout with horseradish sauce (without
 brown bread and butter)
Stuffed vine leaves

200 to 300 Calories
Cream of tomato soup
Cream of watercress soup
Egg Florentine
French onion soup with toasted cheese topping
Globe artichoke with butter
Lobster or crab bisque
Mixed fish salad (*insalata di mare*)

Starters

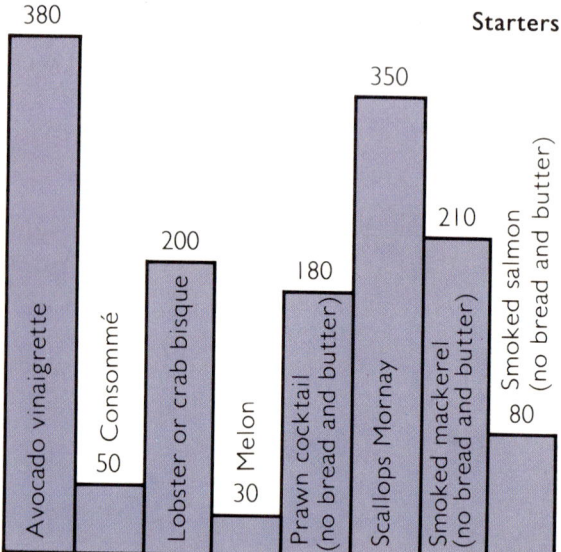

Smoked mackerel (without bread and butter)
Spring roll

300 to 400 Calories
Avocado with prawns
Avocado vinaigrette
Corn on the cob with butter
Cream of mushroom soup
Humus with pitta bread
Pâté with toast
Scallops Mornay
Scallops Parisienne
Spaghetti Bolognese
Whitebait

400 Calories and over
Cannelloni
Chinese spare ribs
Fried scampi with tartare sauce
Lasagne verdi
Mixed hors d'oeuvre
Taramasalata with pitta bread

Main courses

Under 300 Calories
Beef salad (no dressing)
Braised kidneys
Cottage cheese and fruit salad (no dressing)
Crab salad (no dressing or seafood sauce)
Fillet steak, well grilled, 175 g/6 oz raw weight
Grilled gammon and pineapple
Grilled halibut
Grilled lobster
Grilled trout
Grilled turbot
Ham salad (no dressing)
Herb omelette or plain omelette
Lobster salad (no dressing or seafood sauce)
Poached halibut (no Hollandaise sauce)
Poached salmon (no Hollandaise sauce)
Poached turbot (no Hollandaise sauce)
Prawn salad (no dressing or seafood sauce)
Rump or sirloin steak, well or medium grilled,
    175 g/6 oz raw weight

Main courses

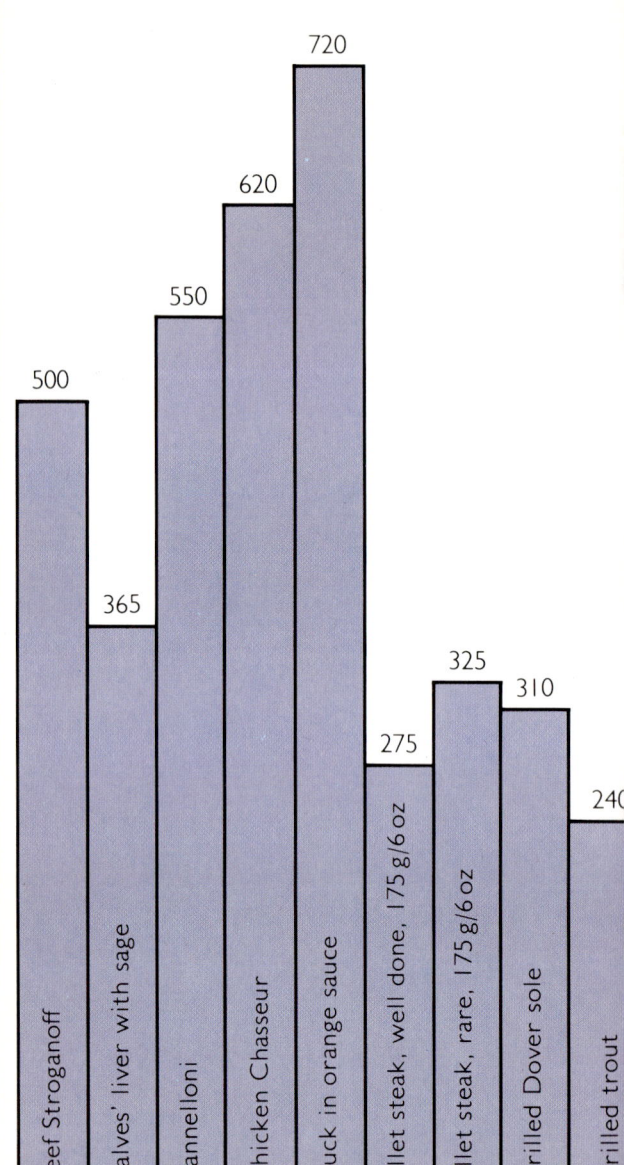

Dish	Calories
Beef Stroganoff	500
Calves' liver with sage	365
Cannelloni	550
Chicken Chasseur	620
Duck in orange sauce	720
Fillet steak, well done, 175 g/6 oz	275
Fillet steak, rare, 175 g/6 oz	325
Grilled Dover sole	310
Grilled trout	240

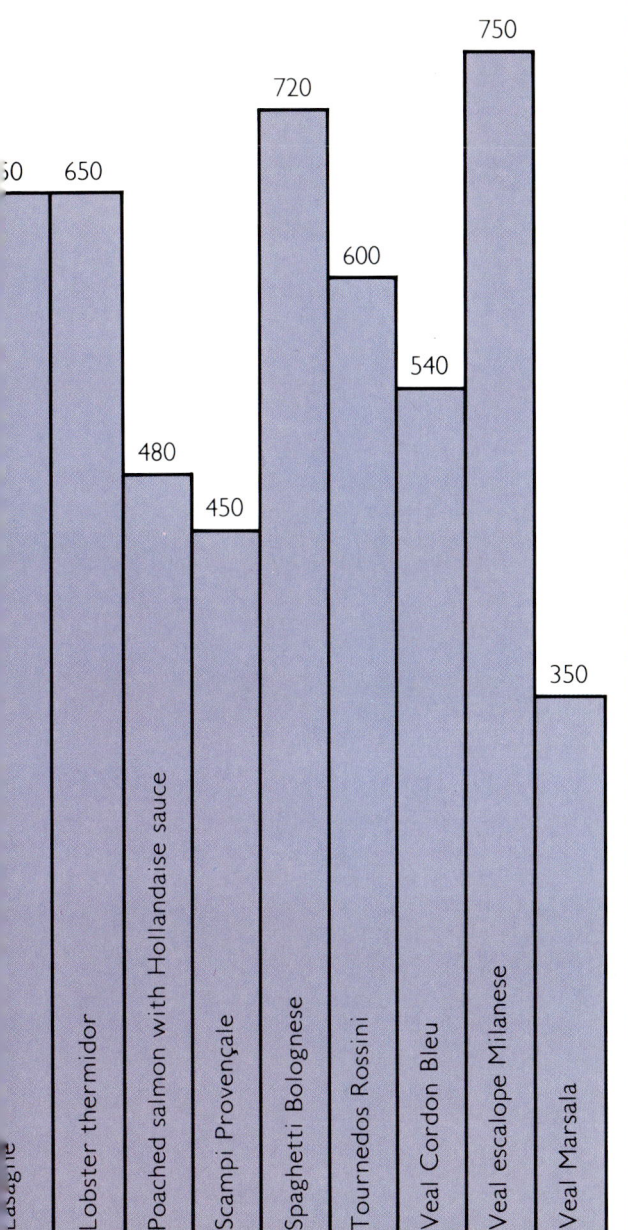

50 650 480 450 720 600 540 750 350

Lobster thermidor
Poached salmon with Hollandaise sauce
Scampi Provençale
Spaghetti Bolognese
Tournedos Rossini
Veal Cordon Bleu
Veal escalope Milanese
Veal Marsala

Salmon salad (no dressing or mayonnaise)
Trout au bleu

300 to 400 Calories

Calves' liver with sage
Cheese salad (no dressing)
Fillet steak, rare grilled, 175 g/6 oz raw weight
Fillet steak, medium or well grilled, 225 g/8 oz raw
 weight
Grilled Dover sole
Grilled salmon
Ham omelette
Kidneys Turbigo
Lamb kebabs
Mixed fish salad
Roast beef, Yorkshire pudding and gravy
Roast chicken and trimmings
Roast pork, apple sauce and gravy
Rump or sirloin steak, rare grilled, 175 g/6 oz raw
 weight
Rump or sirloin steak, well or medium grilled,
 225 g/8 oz raw weight
Skate with black butter
Steak Tartare
Tandoori chicken
Trout Meunière
Veal Marsala

400 to 500 Calories

Beef Stroganoff
Carbonnade of beef
Cheese omelette
Chilli con carne
Cod or haddock Mornay
Fillet steak, rare grilled, 225 g/8 oz raw weight
Escalope of veal fried in breadcrumbs
King prawn curry
Liver and bacon
Plaice fried in breadcrumbs
Poached halibut with Hollandaise sauce
Poached salmon with Hollandaise sauce
Poached turbot with Hollandaise sauce
Rump or sirloin steak, rare grilled, 225 g/8 oz raw
 weight
72 Salmon mayonnaise

Scampi Provençale
Sole Meunière
Trout with almonds
Turbot with shrimp or prawn sauce
Vegetable curry

500 to 600 Calories
Beef olives
Beef in red wine
Cannelloni
Chicken pie
Escalope of veal Holstein
Fried scampi with tartare sauce
Goujons of plaice with tartare sauce
Meat madras
Mixed grill
Sole Bercy
Sole Bonne Femme
Sole Portuguaise
Sole Véronique
Steak and kidney pie
Veal Cordon Bleu

600 to 700 Calories
Beef Wellington
Chicken Chasseur
Chicken Marengo
Chicken Véronique
Coq au vin
Lasagne
Lobster thermidor
Paella
Steak and kidney pudding
Steak Diane
Tournedos Rossini

Over 700 calories
Chicken Korma
Chicken Maryland
Duck in orange sauce
Fritto misto
Moussaka
Pizza
Spaghetti Bolognese
Veal escalope Milanese

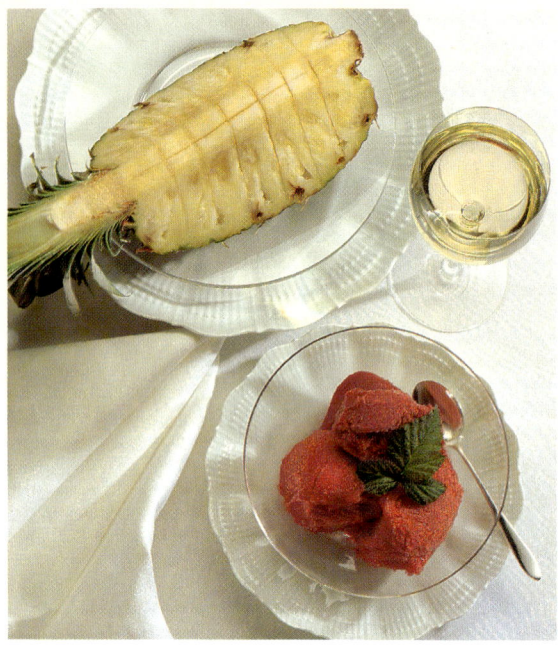

ABOVE: Pineapple with Kirsch and sorbet.

Desserts

Do not add extra cream to any of the desserts.

Under 100 calories
Canned lychees
Fresh fruit
Fresh raspberries with sugar
Fresh strawberries with sugar
Pineapple with Kirsch
Sorbet

100 to 200 Calories
Cassata
Crême caramel
Fresh fruit salad
Ice cream with wafer
Orange in caramel
Pancakes with lemon and sugar
Peaches Cardinal

Peach Melba
Pears in red wine
Zabaglione with sponge finger

200 to 300 Calories
Bread and butter pudding
Chocolate mousse
Coupe Jacques
Fruit flan
Grand Marnier soufflé (hot)
Ice cream sundae with sauce and nuts
Lemon soufflé (cold) or lemon mousse
Orange soufflé (cold) or orange mousse
Pears Belle Hélène
Summer pudding

300 to 400 Calories
Apple strudel
Black Forest gâteau
Crêpes Suzette
Meringue gâteau with fruit and cream
Raspberries with sugar and cream
Sponge gâteau with fruit and cream
Strawberries with sugar and cream
Syllabub

400 to 500 Calories
Cheesecake
Chocolate soufflé (hot)
Jam roly poly (no custard)
Lemon meringue pie
Rum baba
Savarin
Spotted Dick (no custard)

Over 500 Calories
Apple pie and cream, custard or ice cream
Chocolate meringue gâteau
Chocolate profiteroles
Christmas pudding with brandy butter or cream
Jam roly poly and custard
Millefeuille
Spotted Dick and custard
Treacle tart and custard
Trifle

Vegetables and salads

The calories in this chart are for an average portion of vegetables served in a restaurant. They are higher in calories than in the basic chart on page 41 because we have allowed for the extras such as butter, oil and sugar that chefs usually add. If additions are minimal, calories could be slightly lower; but if the chef is generous with butter or oil, calories per portion may well be higher.

Hot vegetables
Per average portion:

Asparagus	60
Broad beans	70
Broccoli	50
Brussels sprouts	50
Brussels sprouts with chestnuts	150
Cabbage	50
Cabbage, red with apples	70
Carrots	50
Cauliflower	20
Cauliflower with cheese sauce	150
Courgettes, sautéed	60
French beans or haricots verts	60
Jerusalem artichokes	50
Leeks	50
Leeks in white sauce	150
Mushrooms, fried, as a garnish	80
Mushrooms, fried, as a vegetable	160
Onion rings, fried in batter	270
Onions, button, glazed	50
Onions, sliced, fried	50
Parsnips, roast	120
Peas	70
Petits pois à la Française	120
Potatoes, Anna	250
Potatoes, boiled, new	160
Potatoes, Boulangère	260
Potatoes, chips	350
Potatoes, creamed	260
Potatoes, jacket baked	200
Potatoes, jacket baked with butter	300
Potatoes, jacket baked with soured cream	260
Potatoes, roast, 2 medium	150

Potatoes, sautéed	200
Ratatouille	80
Spinach	60
Tomatoes, raw, each	10
Tomatoes, grilled, each	20

Salads

Coleslaw	200
Green salad without dressing	15
Green salad with dressing	100
Mixed salad without dressing	20
Mixed salad with dressing	100
Potato salad	350
Tomato and onion salad without dressing	20
Tomato and onion salad with dressing	100

Vegetables and salads

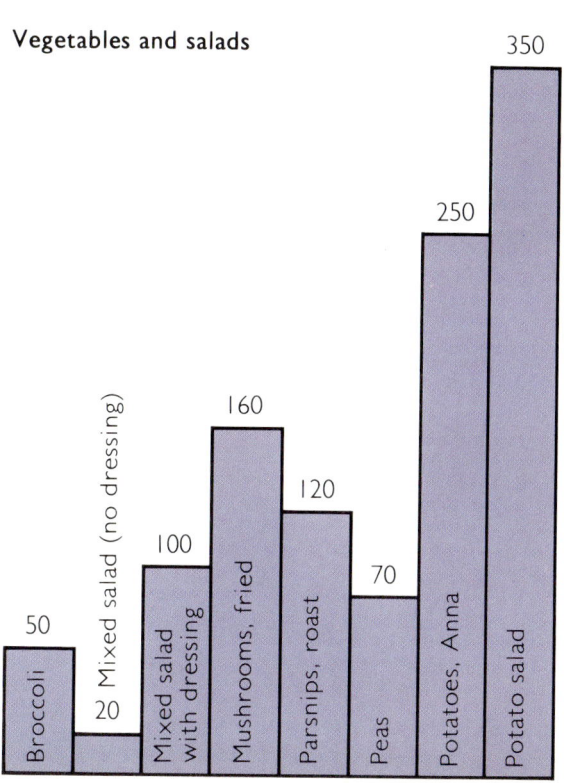

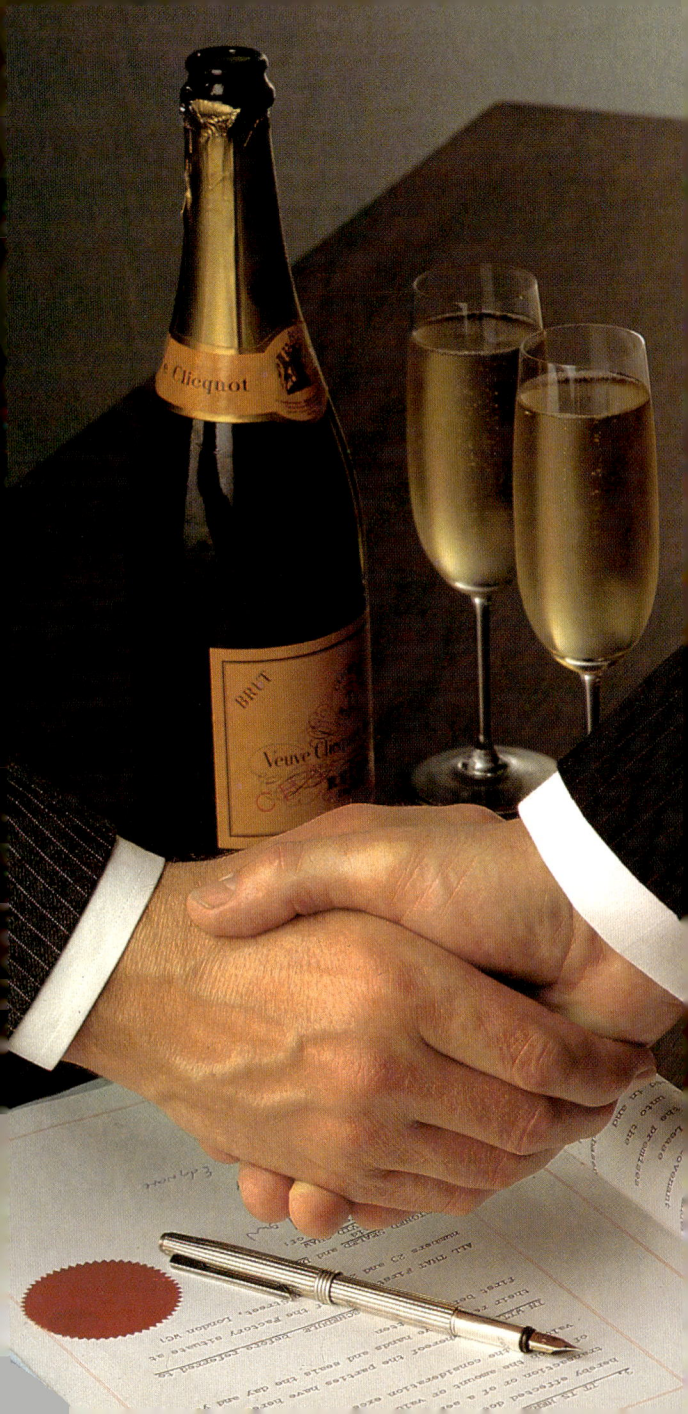

ALCOHOLIC DRINKS

If the drinking man gave up his daily tipples, it could well be enough to lose him pounds without any other dieting. But sometimes it isn't considered socially acceptable for a man to sit and sip a low-calorie tonic water. Alcoholic drinks contain few nutrients, so it is best to keep drink calories as a minor part of your total allowance. Experts also warn that heavy drinking can cause health problems, so moderation is best for your body in both respects.

Here's a guide to what your alcoholic drink will cost you in calories, either in the pub or at home.

Calorie cutters

* Spirits are higher in calories than wines, but are drunk in smaller quantities. A single gin and low-calorie tonic will cost you less than a glass of wine.
* As a general rule, the stronger the beer, the higher it is in calories. If you want the taste rather than the alcohol, cut some calories by choosing a non-alcoholic lager from the list on page 93. Don't make the mistake of thinking that low-carbohydrate or diabetic lagers are low in calories, though – usually they are not.
* If you are thirsty, start off with a low-calorie mixer, a mineral water, or a lime cordial filled up with soda water. Never quench a thirst with an alcoholic drink – save that for sipping and savouring.

Cinzano

Per pub measure, 50 ml/$\frac{1}{3}$ gill, unless otherwise stated:

Cinzano Bianco	80
Cinzano Bianco, per 15 ml tablespoon	25

Cinzano Bianco with low-calorie lemonade	85
Cinzano Bianco with ½ small bottle ordinary lemonade	100
Cinzano Rosso	75
Cinzano Rosso, per 15 ml tablespoon	25
Cinzano Rosso with soda water	75

Martini

Per pub measure, 50 ml/⅓ gill, unless otherwise stated:

Martini Bianco	95
Martini Bianco with low-calorie lemonade	100
Martini Bianco with ½ small bottle ordinary bitter lemon	120
Martini Bianco, Rosé and Rosso, per 15 ml tablespoon	25
Martini Extra Dry	65
Martini Extra Dry with low-calorie lemonade	70
Martini Rosé	90
Martini Rosso	95
Martini Rosso with low-calorie lemonade	100
Martini Rosso with ½ small bottle ordinary bitter lemon	120

Dubonnet

Per pub measure, 50 ml/⅓ gill, unless otherwise stated:

Dubonnet Dry	55
Dubonnet Dry, per 15 ml tablespoon	15
Dubonnet Dry, with low-calorie lemonade	60
Dubonnet Red	75
Dubonnet Red, per 15 ml tablespoon	25
Dubonnet Red with diet cola	75
Dubonnet Red with soda	75

Riccadonna

Per pub measure, 50 ml/⅓ gill, unless otherwise stated:

Riccadonna Bianco Vermouth	80
Riccadonna Bianco Vermouth, per 15 ml tablespoon	25

Riccadonna Bianco Vermouth with
low-calorie lemonade 85
Riccadonna Bianco Vermouth with $\frac{1}{2}$ small
bottle ordinary lemonade 100
Riccadonna Extra Dry Vermouth 50
Riccadonna Extra Dry Vermouth, per 15 ml
tablespoon 15
Riccadonna Extra Dry Vermouth with
low-calorie tonic water 60
Riccadonna Rosé Vermouth 75
Riccadonna Rosé Vermouth, per 15 ml
tablespoon 25
Riccadonna Rosé Vermouth with soda water 75
Riccadonna Rosso Vermouth 80
Riccadonna Rosso Vermouth, per 15 ml
tablespoon 25
Riccadonna Rosso Vermouth with
low-calorie lemonade 85
Riccadonna Rosso Vermouth with $\frac{1}{2}$ small
bottle ordinary lemonade 100

Campari

Per pub measure, 50 ml/$\frac{1}{3}$ gill, unless otherwise
stated:
Campari 115
Campari, per 15 ml tablespoon 35
Campari with soda water 115
Campari with 1 small bottle ordinary
lemonade 155

Pernod

Per pub measure, 25 ml/$\frac{1}{6}$ gill:
Pernod 65
Pernod with low-calorie lemonade 70
Pernod with 25 ml/1 fl oz undiluted
blackcurrant cordial 95

Light ale

Per 284 ml/$\frac{1}{2}$ pint unless otherwise stated:
Home-brewed, average value 120
Toby, 275 ml/9.7 fl oz bottle 70
Whitbread 75

Bitter and brown ale

Per 284 ml/½ pint unless otherwise stated:

Courage Brown Ale, 275 ml/9.7 fl oz can or bottle	85
Draught Bitter, average value	90
Forest Brown	85
Home-brewed bitter or brown ale, average value	120
Newcastle Brown Ale, 440 ml/15.5 fl oz can	175
Stones Bitter	90
Tartan Bitter, 440 ml/15.5 fl oz can	115
Toby Brown Ale, 275 ml/9.7 fl oz bottle	70

Stout

Per 284 ml/½ pint unless otherwise stated:

Draught Guinness	90
Guinness Extra	100
Mackeson Stout	115
Younger's Sweet Stout, 275 ml/9.7 fl oz bottle	60

Strong beers

Per 284 ml/½ pint unless otherwise stated:

Fullers Golden Pride	225
Fullers London Pride	105
Fullers Strong Ale	180
Ind Coope Long Life	100
Newcastle Amber Ale, 275 ml/9.7 fl oz bottle	70
Ruddles Country Strong Bitter	120
Tartan Special, 440 ml/15.5 fl oz can	115
Watneys Red	70
Watneys Special	70
Whitbread Brewmaster	110
Whitbread English Ale	105

Lager

Per 284 ml/½ pint, unless otherwise stated:

Arctic Lite Lager	80
Carling Black Label	95
Carlsberg '68, 330 ml/11 fl oz	185
Carlsberg De Luxe, 275 ml/9.7 fl oz	125
Carlsberg Export Hof	110

Carlsberg Pilsner, 275 ml/9.7 fl oz	75
Carlsberg Special Brew	205
Export Hof	110
Harp	80
Heineken	85
Heldenbrau, 275 ml/9.7 fl oz bottle	70
Hemeling	80
Henninger Diet Pils, 275 ml/9.7 fl oz	100
Hofmeister, 275 ml/9.7 fl oz can	85
Hofmeister	95
Holstein Pils Diabetic, 270 ml/9.5 fl oz bottle	105
Kaltenberg Diät Pils	115
Kronenbourg, 275 ml/9.7 fl oz can	110
Lamot Pilsor Strong Lager, per 275 ml/ 9.7 fl oz bottle	105
Lite, 275 ml/9.7 fl oz	85
McEwan's, 440 ml/15.5 fl oz can	130
Satzenbrau	110
Skol	90
Stella Artois	120
Tennent's	95
Tennent's Extra	110
Tennent's Pilsner	85
Younger's Kestrel, 440 ml/15.5 fl oz can	110

Cider

Per 284 ml/$\frac{1}{2}$ pint unless otherwise stated:	
Bulmers Conditioned Draught, dry	85
Bulmers Conditioned Draught, medium	80
Bulmers Conditioned Draught, sweet	95
Bulmers No 7	100
Bulmers Original	105
Bulmers Perry	120
Bulmers Pomagne, dry	150
Bulmers Pomagne, sweet	185
Bulmers Special Cellar	160
Bulmers Special Reserve, dry	135
Bulmers Special Reserve, medium sweet	160
Bulmers Strongbow	100
Bulmers West Country Still Draught, dry	95
Bulmers West Country Still Draught, extra dry	90
Bulmers West Country Still Draught, medium	110

Bulmers West Country Still Draught, sweet	115
Bulmers Woodpecker	80
Bulmers Woodpecker, dry	85
Bulmers Woodpecker, still	95
Bulmers Woodpecker Keg Draught	100
Coates Farmhouse	150
Coates Festival VAT	135
Coates Scrumpy	125
Coates Somerset	90
Coates Triple Vintage	180
Gaymers Lite, 275 ml/9.5 fl oz bottle	75
Gaymers Norfolk Dry, 275 ml/9.5 fl oz bottle	105
Gaymers Old English, 275 ml/9.5 fl oz bottle	115
Gaymers Pommetta, dry, 115 ml/4 fl oz	60
Gaymers Pommetta, sweet, 115 ml/4 fl oz	75
La Cidroie, 250 ml/8 fl oz bottle	80
Taunton Autumn Gold, 275 ml/9.7 fl oz bottle	95
Taunton Dry Blackthorn, 275 ml/9.7 fl oz bottle	95
Taunton Exhibition, dry	150
Taunton Exhibition, sweet	180
Taunton Pommia, dry	155
Taunton Pommia, sweet	190
Taunton Special VAT, 275 ml/9.7 fl oz bottle	110
Trumpet, 142 ml/$\frac{1}{4}$ pint	80

Wines

The following calorie counts give an average assessment for all wines in the various categories.
Per average glass, 115 ml/4 fl oz:

Champagne	85
De-alcoholized wines	30
Dry red	80
Dry white	75
Rosé	80
Sparkling white	85
Sweet red	95
Sweet white	105

Per 150 ml/5 fl oz glass:

Champagne	110
De-alcoholized wines	35
Dry red	95
Dry white	95
Rosé	100

Sparkling white	110
Sweet red	120
Sweet white	135

Port

Average values for all brands, per pub measure,
50 ml/$\frac{1}{3}$ gill, unless otherwise stated:

Port	75
Port and 175 ml/6 fl oz bottle low-calorie lemonade	80
Port and $\frac{1}{2}$ small bottle ordinary lemonade	100

Sherry

Per small schooner, 50 ml/$\frac{1}{3}$ gill:

Cream	65
Dry	55
Medium	60

Per 15 ml tablespoon:

Cream	20
Dry	15
Medium	20

Liqueurs

Per pub measure, 25 ml/$\frac{1}{6}$ gill:

Advocaat	65
Bailey's Original Irish Cream	85
Bénédictine	90
Calvados	60
Chartreuse, green	100
Cherry Brandy	60
Cointreau	85
Crème de Cassis	65
Crème de Menthe	80
Drambuie	85
Galliano	75
Grand Marnier	80
Kirsch	50
Kümmel	75
Malibu	50
Strega	75
Tia Maria	75

Alcoholic drinks

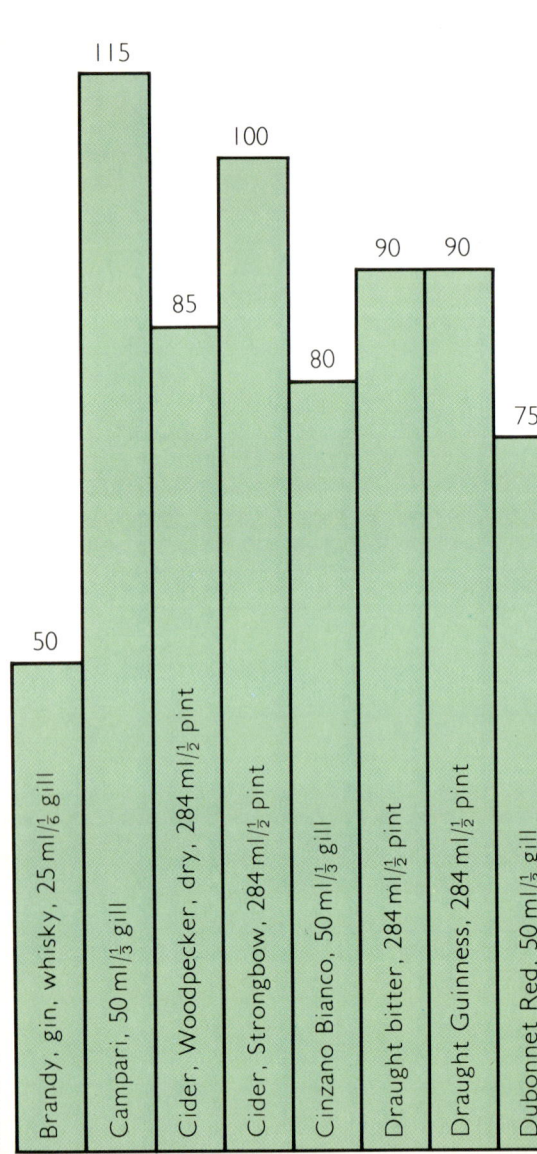

50	Brandy, gin, whisky, 25 ml/$\frac{1}{6}$ gill
115	Campari, 50 ml/$\frac{1}{3}$ gill
85	Cider, Woodpecker, dry, 284 ml/$\frac{1}{2}$ pint
100	Cider, Strongbow, 284 ml/$\frac{1}{2}$ pint
80	Cinzano Bianco, 50 ml/$\frac{1}{3}$ gill
90	Draught bitter, 284 ml/$\frac{1}{2}$ pint
90	Draught Guinness, 284 ml/$\frac{1}{2}$ pint
75	Dubonnet Red, 50 ml/$\frac{1}{3}$ gill
80	Grand Marnier, 25 ml/$\frac{1}{2}$ gill

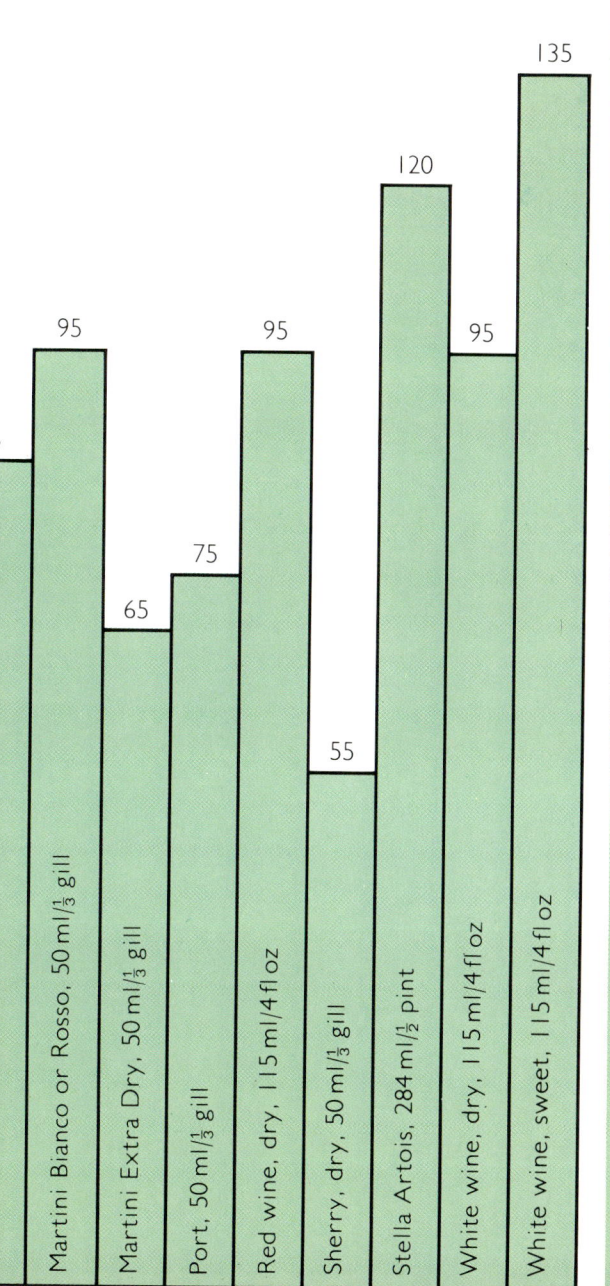

5

95 Martini Bianco or Rosso, 50 ml/⅓ gill

65 Martini Extra Dry, 50 ml/⅓ gill

75 Port, 50 ml/⅓ gill

95 Red wine, dry, 115 ml/4 fl oz

55 Sherry, dry, 50 ml/⅓ gill

120 Stella Artois, 284 ml/½ pint

95 White wine, dry, 115 ml/4 fl oz

135 White wine, sweet, 115 ml/4 fl oz

Spirits

Per pub measure, 25 ml/$\frac{1}{6}$ gill unless otherwise stated:

Brandy	50
Brandy, per 15 ml tablespoon	30
Brandy and low-calorie lemonade	55
Gin	50
Gin, per 15 ml tablespoon	30
Gin and low-calorie tonic water	60
Gin and 113 ml/4 fl oz bottle unsweetened orange juice	95
Ouzo	60
Ouzo with low-calorie lemonade	65
Ouzo with 1 small bottle ordinary lemonade	110
Rum	50
Rum, per 15 ml tablespoon	30
Rum and diet cola	50
Rum and 25 ml/1 fl oz undiluted blackcurrant cordial	80
Tequila	50
Tequila, per 15 ml tablespoon	30
Tequila, and 25 ml/1 fl oz undiluted lime cordial	75
Vodka	50
Vodka, per 15 ml tablespoon	30
Vodka and low-calorie tonic water	60
Vodka and 113 ml/4 fl oz bottle tomato juice or tomato juice cocktail	75
Vodka and 113 ml/4 fl oz bottle unsweetened orange juice	95
Whisky, (Scotch, Irish or Bourbon)	50
Whisky, per 15 ml tablespoon	30
Whisky and low-calorie American ginger ale	55
Whisky and soda	50

Shaker's cocktails

Per 160 ml/5.3 fl oz bottle:

Bananarama	245
Margarita	175
New Yorker	175
Pina Colada	235
Sundowner	180

Other alcoholic drinks

Per standard bottle:

Babycham, dry	60
Babycham, sweet	80
Cherry B	140
Crocodillo	60
Goldwell's Calypso	100
Goldwell's Wee McGlen	100
Phosphenne Tonic Wine, 150 ml/5 fl oz	200
Pimm's No 1 Cup, 50 ml/$\frac{1}{3}$ gill, with low-calorie lemonade	100
Pony	130

Calorie cutters

★ It is very easy to pour a double or even a treble measure of spirits at home if you just tip the bottle straight into the glass. A set of optic measures are a good diet aid. Alternatively, you can use a 15 ml measuring spoon and you'll find tablespoon calories in the chart.

★ Serve drinks on the rocks – the ice will melt and make your drink last longer with no more calories. Although sherry and liqueurs are usually served neat, you can make more of them by adding soda water or a low-calorie mixer.

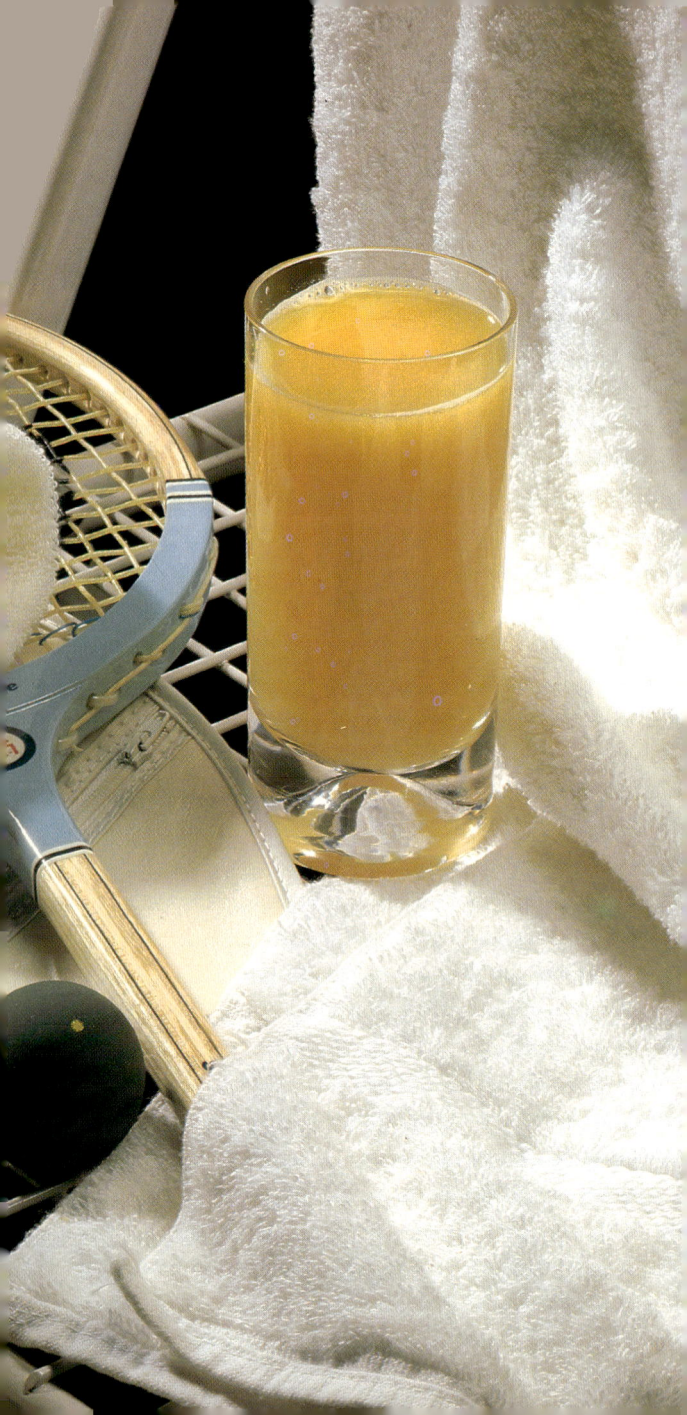

NON-ALCOHOLIC DRINKS

If your weight loss is not as speedy as you would wish, take a special look at what you are drinking. It is very easy to forget that drink calories count, especially when they have such innocent sounding names as orange or apple juice. If at the end of the day your waste paper basket is full of empty lemonade cans or empty fruit juice cartons, you could be consuming literally hundreds of drink calories. Check the charts below, and make sure you keep these calories under control.

Calorie cutters

★ Low-calorie mixers are a boon to slimmers. On a 170 ml/6 fl oz bottle of bitter lemon, for instance, the saving is 50 Calories if you choose a low-calorie brand rather than the ordinary sort.

★ Half fill a long glass with unsweetened fruit juice and top up with sparkling mineral water or soda. This refreshing fruit drink will cost around 75 Calories.

★ Be adventurous with tea. A delicately flavoured tea, such as Earl Grey, is delicious served with a slice of lemon. Mint tea is very refreshing on a hot day. No tea will cost you any calories worth counting unless you add milk or sugar.

Fruit juices

Apple, unsweetened, per 275 ml/½ pint	100
Grapefruit, sweetened, per 275 ml/½ pint	110
Grapefruit, sweetened, per pub bottle, 113 ml/4 fl oz	45
Grapefruit, unsweetened, per 275 ml/½ pint	90
Orange, sweetened, per 275 ml/½ pint	140
Orange, sweetened, per pub bottle, 113 ml/4 fl oz	55

Orange, unsweetened, per 275 ml/½ pint	110
Orange, unsweetened, per pub bottle, 113 ml/4 fl oz	45
Pineapple, unsweetened, per 275 ml/½ pint	150
Pineapple, unsweetened, per pub bottle, 113 ml/4 fl oz	60
Tomato, per 275 ml/½ pint	60
Tomato or tomato cocktail, per pub bottle, 113 ml/4 fl oz	25

Mixers and carbonated drinks

Per medium bottle or can:	
American ginger ale, 180 ml/6.3 fl oz	60
Bitter lemon, 180 ml/6.3 fl oz	65
Coca Cola, 330 ml/11.6 fl oz	130
Diet Coke, 330 ml/11.6 fl oz	0
Diet Pepsi, 330 ml/11.6 fl oz	0

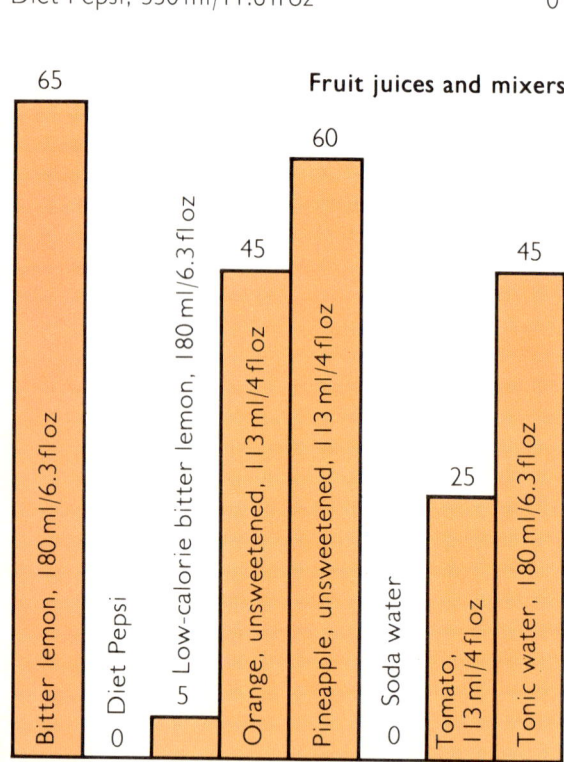

Fruit juices and mixers

65 — Bitter lemon, 180 ml/6.3 fl oz
0 — Diet Pepsi
5 — Low-calorie bitter lemon, 180 ml/6.3 fl oz
45 — Orange, unsweetened, 113 ml/4 fl oz
60 — Pineapple, unsweetened, 113 ml/4 fl oz
0 — Soda water
25 — Tomato, 113 ml/4 fl oz
45 — Tonic water, 180 ml/6.3 fl oz

Dry ginger ale, 180 ml/6.3 fl oz	35
Ginger beer, 180 ml/6.3 fl oz	75
Lemonade, 330 ml/11.6 fl oz	90
Low-calorie American ginger ale	5
Low-calorie bitter lemon, 180 ml/6.3 fl oz	5
Low-calorie lemonade, 330 ml/11.6 fl oz	10
Low-calorie tonic water, 180 ml/6.3 fl oz	10
Lucozade, 250 ml/8.8 fl oz	180
Mineral water	0
Pepsi Cola, 330 ml/11.6 fl oz	145
Soda water, 180 ml/6.3 fl oz	0
Tonic water, 180 ml/6.3 fl oz	45

Non-alcoholic lagers

Barbican, 275 ml/9.7 fl oz bottle	40
Claysthaler Special Lager, 330 ml/11.3 fl oz bottle	90
Danish Light, 320 ml/11 fl oz can	55
Sainsbury's Non-Alcoholic Lager, per bottle	90
St Christopher, 275 ml/9.7 fl oz bottle	40

Squashes and cordials

Per 28 ml/1 fl oz, undiluted:

All flavours	30
Low-calorie, all flavours	5

Milk and milk drinks

Per 275 ml/$\frac{1}{2}$ pint unless otherwise stated:

Banana-flavoured low-fat milk	170
Channel Island or Gold Top	225
Chocolate-flavoured low-fat milk	190
Evaporated, per 15 ml/1 tablespoon	25
Long Life (UHT)	190
Semi-skimmed	150
Silver Top or whole milk	190
Skimmed	100
Skimmed, powdered, per 10 ml/1 rounded teaspoon	15
Strawberry-flavoured low-fat milk	165

Milkshakes

Per average thick milkshake:

McDonalds Chocolate Shake	385
McDonalds Strawberry Shake	360
McDonalds Vanilla Shake	350
Wimpy shake, any flavour	260

Hot beverages

Per average cup, 150 ml/¼ pint. All beverages are unsweetened. Add artificial sweetener if required.

Coffee, black	0
Coffee, with dash of skimmed milk	10
Coffee, with dash of whole cold milk	20
Coffee, made with half water and half hot milk	45
Coffee, with single cream	60
Drinking chocolate, made with water and a dash of skimmed milk	55
Drinking chocolate, made with skimmed milk	95
Drinking chocolate, made with whole milk	140

Hot drinks

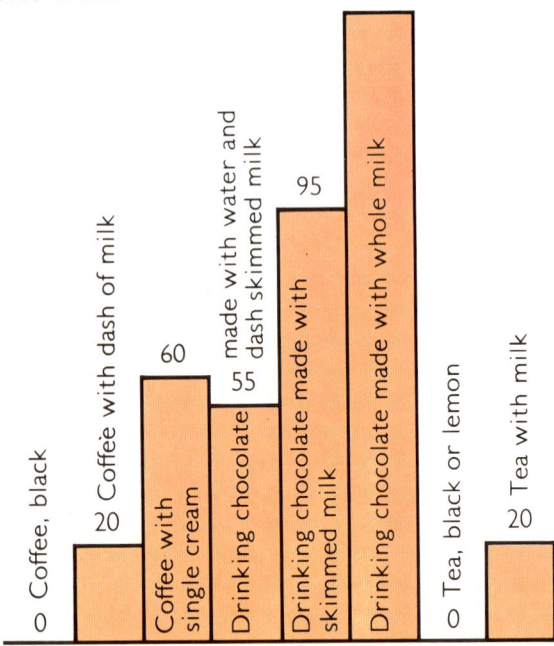

140 — Drinking chocolate made with whole milk
95 — Drinking chocolate made with skimmed milk
60 — Coffee with dash of milk
55 — Drinking chocolate made with water and dash skimmed milk
20 — Coffee with single cream
20 — Tea with milk
0 — Coffee, black
0 — Tea, black or lemon

Malted milk bedtime drink, made with water and a dash of skimmed milk	65
Malted milk bedtime drink, made with skimmed milk	105
Malted milk bedtime drink, made with whole milk	150
Tea, black or lemon	0
Tea, with skimmed milk	10
Tea, with whole milk	20

Dispenser drinks

Maxpax vending machine drinks

Per cup:

Blackcurrant	25
Chicken soup	25
Chocolate	65
Coffee, black with sugar	25
Coffee, white, no sugar	25
Lemon drink	25
Lemon tea	35
Orange	25
Oxtail soup	25
Tea, with dash milk	10
Tea, white	20
Tomato soup	20
Vegetable soup	25

Drinkmaster vending machine drinks

Per cup:

Blackcurrant	30
Bovril	15
Chicken soup	30
Chocolate-flavoured drink	55
Coffee, decaffeinated, white	30
Coffee, white, no sugar	15
Coffee, white, with sugar	40
Lemon drink	60
Lemon tea	40
Orange	55
Oxtail soup	35
Tea, white, with sugar	40
Tea, white, no sugar	10
Tomato soup	30
Vegetable soup	25

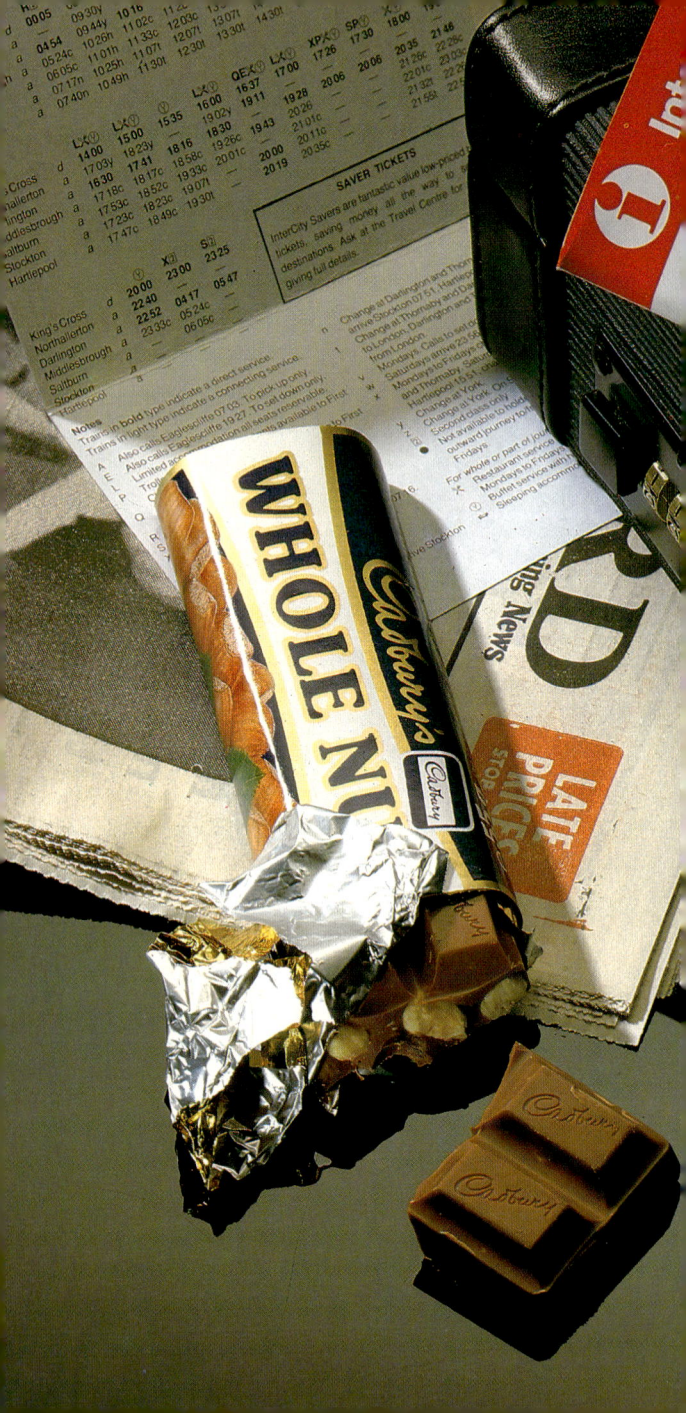

TRAVEL SNACKS

You may like to buy a chocolate bar to munch on the train home or to eat in the car when driving between appointments. This is fine as long as you count the calories into your daily total.

Chocolate and sweets

Per bar unless otherwise stated:

Aero, chunky size bar	170
Aero, standard shape, any flavour	210
Bounty, twin bar	300
Cadbury Crunchie	165
Cadbury Dairy Milk, 40 g/1½ oz	210
Cadbury Flake	180
Cadbury Fruit and Nut, 57 g/2 oz	270
Cadbury Whole Nut, 53 g/1⅞ oz	305
Chewing gum, per stick	10
Fruit gums, per roll	55
Fry's Peppermint Cream Bar	210
Fry's Turkish Delight	185
Kit Kat, 4 fingers	250
Mars Bar	330
Milk Yorkie	320
Peanut Yorkie	300
Polo Fruits, per roll	105
Polo Mints, per roll	95
Rolo, per tube	225
Rowntree's Toffee Crisp	225
Rowntree's Walnut Whip	170
Terry's Chocolate Waifa Bar	175
Twix Bar, twin bar	270

Crisps and nuts

Crisps, any flavour, 30 g/1⅛ oz packet	150
Dry roasted cashews, 50 g/1¾ oz pack	220
Dry roasted peanuts, 50 g/1¾ oz pack	280
Nuts and raisins, 50 g/1¾ oz pack	245
Salted cashews, 50 g/1¾ oz pack	280
Salted peanuts, 50 g/1¾ oz pack	285

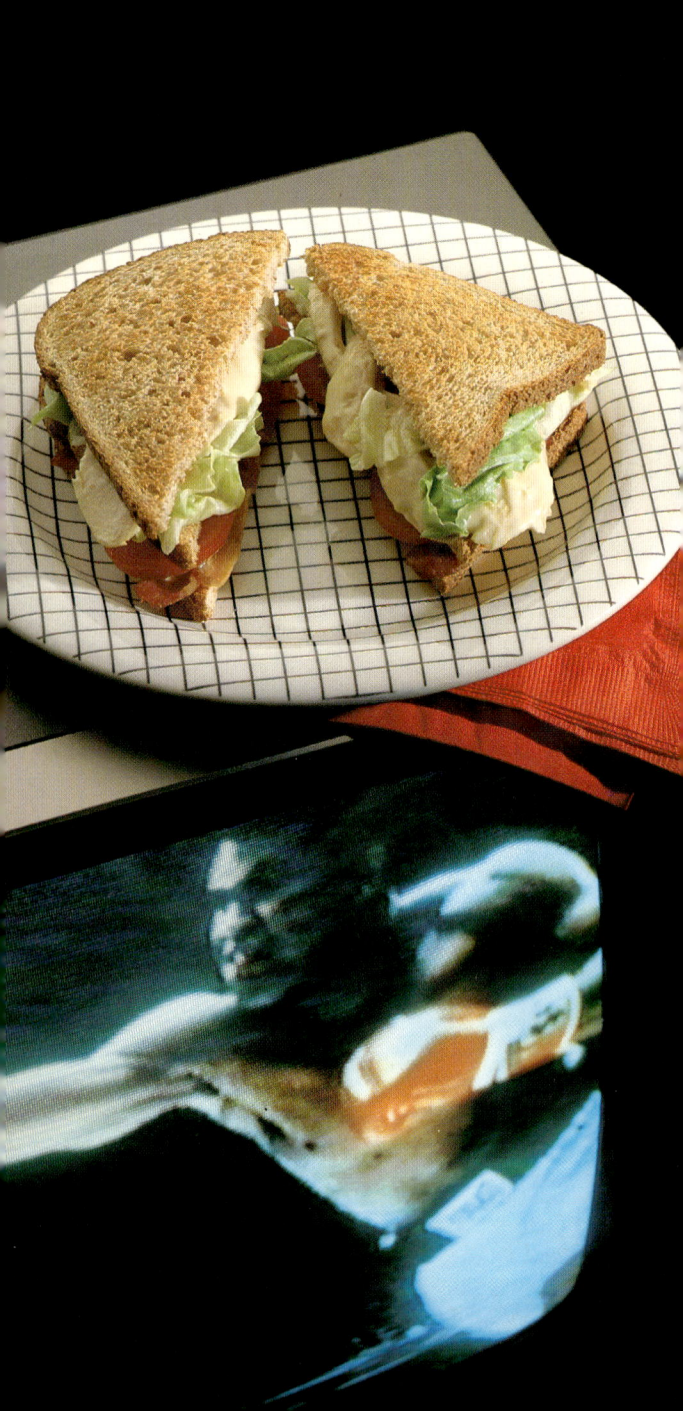

BACHELOR MEALS

Choose your main meal from this section if you are eating alone. They can all be doubled if you want to share, but they have all been devised to take the minimum amount of preparation and cooking. All the meals total 500 Calories, and if you like to end with something sweet, choose some fresh fruit from the list on page 65.

from the list on page 65.

Calorie cutters

★ A green or mixed salad would make a good, low-calorie accompaniment to most main dishes, but calories quickly mount up as soon as you add French dressing. Choosing an oil-free type can save you 70 Calories per 15 ml tablespoon.

★ Top jacket potatoes with low-fat natural yogurt instead of butter and save 95 Calories for every 15 ml tablespoon.

★ If you don't own a non-stick pan, it's worth investing in one. The non-stick surface allows you to cook with a minimum of fat.

Club sandwich with chicken and bacon
500 Calories

50 g/2 oz cooked chicken, skinned and chopped
15 ml/1 level tablespoon low-calorie salad
   dressing
2 rashers streaky bacon, grilled until crisp
1 small tomato, sliced
3 × 40 g/1½ oz slices wholemeal bread, toasted
1 lettuce leaf, shredded

Mix the chicken with the salad dressing. Place the bacon and tomato on 1 slice of toast. Place another slice on top and cover with lettuce and chicken. Top with a slice of toast. Cut in half to serve. Serves 1.

Stir-fried pork and vegetables
500 Calories

25 g/1 oz brown or white long-grain rice
15 ml/1 tablespoon cooking oil
125 g/4 oz lean pork fillet, trimmed of fat and
   diced
200 g/7 oz frozen stir-fry vegetables
5 ml/1 teaspoon soy sauce
salt and pepper

Boil the rice until tender. Drain.

Heat the oil in a non-stick frying pan or wok. Add the pork and stir-fry for 3 minutes. Add the vegetables and stir-fry for another 4 minutes. Add the rice and the soy sauce and season with salt and pepper to taste. Heat through and serve immediately. Serves 1.

Calorie cutter

★ Herbs and spices cost few calories and you can increase amounts given in recipes if you wish.

Liver and bacon with baked beans
500 Calories

125 g/4 oz lamb's or pig's liver, sliced
1.25 ml/$\frac{1}{4}$ teaspoon oil
2 rashers streaky bacon
$\frac{1}{4}$ chicken stock cube
150 ml/$\frac{1}{4}$ pint boiling water
125 g/4 oz button mushrooms
1 × 227 g/8 oz can baked beans in tomato sauce

Brush the liver with the oil and place under a preheated grill for about 5 minutes, or until cooked through, turning once. Meanwhile, grill the bacon until crisp. Crumble the stock cube into a saucepan containing the boiling water and poach the mushrooms over moderate heat for 5 minutes and drain. Heat the baked beans and serve with the liver, bacon and mushrooms. Serves 1.

Gammon and pineapple
500 Calories

175 g/6 oz gammon steak
150 g/5 oz broad beans, fresh, frozen or canned
150 g/5 oz sweetcorn kernels, fresh, frozen or
    canned
1 ring pineapple canned in natural juice, drained
5 ml/1 level teaspoon made mustard or 15 ml/
    1 level tablespoon relish, any flavour

Grill the gammon well. Boil the fresh beans for
about 20 minutes, until tender. Boil the frozen
vegetables according to packet instructions or heat
if canned. Serve the gammon and vegetables with
the pineapple and mustard. Serves 1.

BELOW: Gammon and pineapple.

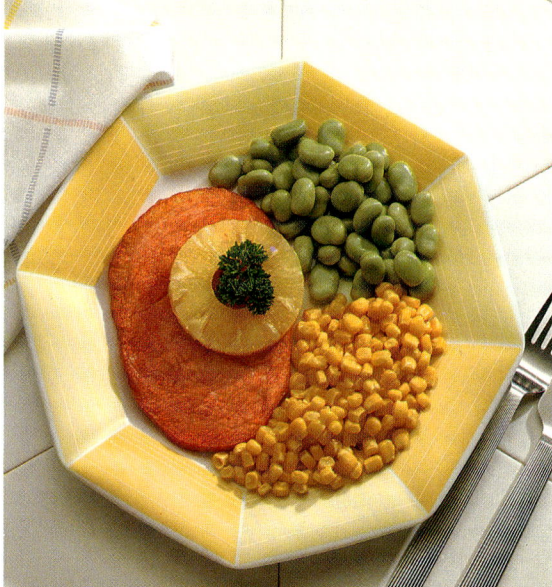

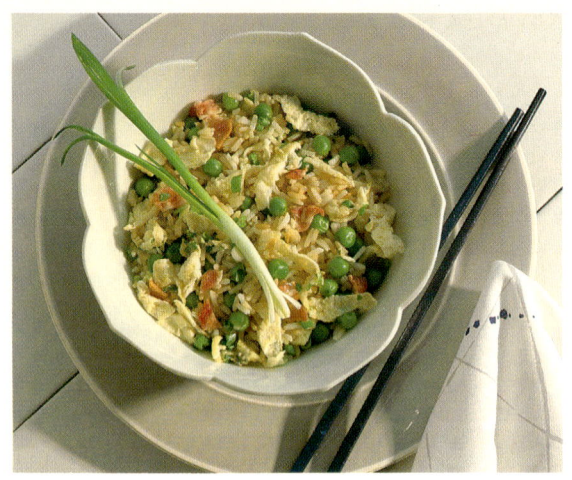

ABOVE: Chinese fried rice.

Chinese fried rice
500 Calories

50 g/2 oz long-grain rice, brown or white
50 g/2 oz frozen peas
1 rasher streaky bacon
1 egg, size 3
salt and pepper
15 ml/1 tablespoon vegetable oil
2 spring onions, chopped
5 ml/1 teaspoon soy sauce

Cook the rice in boiling water until tender. Boil the peas for 5 minutes. Drain the rice and peas and set aside. Grill the bacon until crisp and break into small pieces. In a bowl, lightly beat the egg and season with salt and pepper to taste.

Heat the oil in a non-stick frying pan or wok. Add the spring onions and sauté for 1 to 2 minutes. Add the egg and tilt the pan or wok until the egg covers enough of the surface to make a small omelette. Leave until just set and then stir immediately to break up into small pieces. Add the rice and stir-fry until heated through. Stir in the peas, bacon and soy sauce. Heat through and serve immediately. Serves 1.

Stir-fried beef with beans
500 Calories

15 ml/1 tablespoon vegetable oil
125 g/4 oz lean minced beef
200 g/7 oz frozen stir-fry vegetables
125 g/4 oz cooked or canned red kidney beans, drained
10 ml/2 level teaspoons tomato ketchup
dash of Tabasco sauce
15 ml/1 tablespoon water
salt and pepper

Heat the oil in a non-stick frying pan or wok. Add the beef and stir-fry for 2 minutes. Add the vegetables and stir-fry for another 4 minutes. Add the beans and stir-fry for 1 minute more. Mix the tomato ketchup, Tabasco sauce and water in a small bowl. Stir into the pan and season with salt and pepper. Serve immediately. Serves 1.

Simple chicken risotto
500 Calories

5 ml/1 teaspoon vegetable oil
1 small onion, finely chopped
150 g/5 oz raw boneless chicken breast or 125 g/4 oz cooked chicken, diced
50 g/2 oz long-grain white rice
175 ml/6 fl oz water
$\frac{1}{4}$ chicken stock cube
pinch of dried thyme or mixed herbs
50 g/2 oz mushrooms, chopped
125 g/4 oz frozen mixed vegetables

Heat the oil in a medium saucepan and sauté the onion. Add the raw chicken with the rice, water, stock cube and thyme. Bring to the boil, cover the pan, reduce the heat and simmer gently for 15 minutes.

Add the mushrooms and the mixed vegetables, together with the cooked chicken, if using. Return to the boil, reduce the heat and simmer gently for 10 minutes more. Serves 1.

Cheese omelette
500 Calories

2 tomatoes, halved
2 eggs, size 3
15 ml/1 tablespoon water
25 g/1 oz Cheddar cheese, grated
salt and pepper
7 g/¼ oz butter
1 × 45 g/1¾ oz crusty brown or white bread roll
5 ml/1 level teaspoon low-fat spread

Grill the tomatoes until tender. Meanwhile, beat the eggs lightly with the water in a small bowl. Add half the cheese and season with salt and pepper to taste.

Melt the butter in a small non-stick omelette pan. Pour in the eggs and cook until just set. As the omelette cooks, keep lifting the edges and tilting the pan so that the runny mixture goes underneath. Place the remaining cheese in the centre and fold over. Serve with the tomatoes and the roll spread with low-fat spread. Serves 1.

Lamb chop with jacket potato
500 Calories

1 × 225 g/8 oz potato, scrubbed and pricked
125 g/4 oz carrots, fresh, frozen or canned
125 g/4 oz cauliflower, fresh or frozen
1 × 175 g/6 oz lamb chump chop
5 ml/1 teaspoon mint sauce or 15 ml/1 level
    tablespoon tomato ketchup

Bake the potato in its jacket in a preheated moderately hot oven (200°C/400°F, Gas Mark 6) for about 1 hour or until soft when pinched. Cook the fresh vegetables in separate pans of boiling water until tender – about 20 to 30 minutes. Cook the frozen vegetables according to packet instructions. Heat them if canned. Cook the chop under a preheated grill until well done, about 10 to 15 minutes. Serve with the vegetables and mint sauce or tomato ketchup. Serves 1.

Cheesy fish and vegetables
500 Calories

175 g/6 oz potatoes, weighed peeled
45 ml/3 tablespoons skimmed milk (optional)
salt and pepper
175 g/6 oz cod or haddock fillet
25 g/1 oz Cheddar cheese, grated
15 ml/1 level tablespoon low-calorie salad
  dressing
125 g/4 oz frozen peas

Boil the potatoes until tender. If old, mash with the milk and season with salt and pepper. If new, leave whole.

Meanwhile, cook the fish under a preheated moderate grill until it flakes easily when touched with a fork. Mix the cheese with the salad dressing. Spread on the fish and return to the grill until bubbling.

Cook the peas in a small saucepan with boiling water to cover. Drain and serve with the fish and potatoes. Serves 1.

BELOW: Cheesy fish and vegetables.

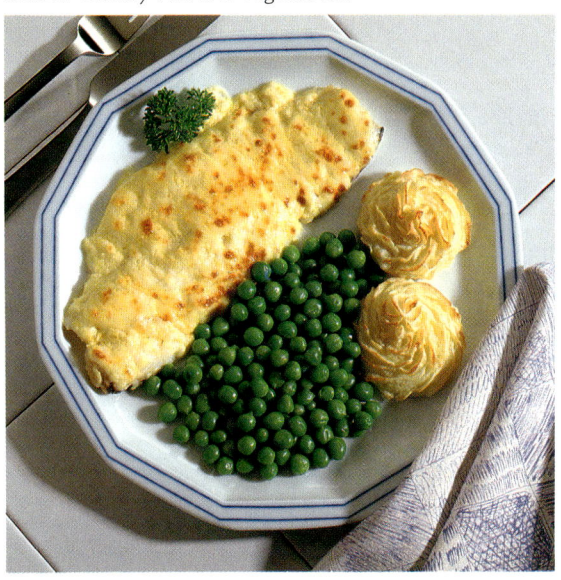

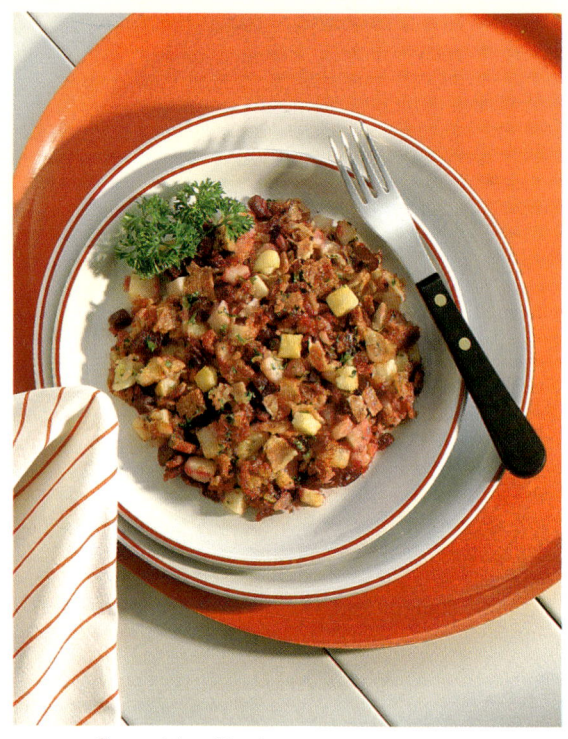

ABOVE: *Corned beef hash.*

Grilled fish and chips
500 Calories

150 g/5 oz frozen grill chips or oven chips
175 g/6 oz plaice, fresh or frozen
5 ml/1 level teaspoon butter
125 g/4 oz frozen peas
15 ml/1 level tablespoon relish, any flavour, or
   tomato ketchup

Cook the chips according to the packet instructions. Dot the fish with the butter and cook under a
preheated moderate grill until it flakes easily when
touched with a fork. Cook the peas in boiling water
for 5 minutes and drain. Serve the fish and vegetables with relish or tomato ketchup. Serves 1.

Corned beef hash
500 Calories

125 g/4 oz potatoes, weighed peeled
10 ml/2 teaspoons vegetable oil
1 small onion, finely chopped
1 rasher streaky bacon, chopped
75 g/3 oz corned beef, chopped
50 g/2 oz boiled beetroot, diced
5 ml/1 level teaspoon chopped fresh parsley or a
  pinch of dried
salt and pepper

Cook the potatoes in boiling water until tender.
Drain and chop them roughly.

Heat the oil in a non-stick frying pan and add the
onion and bacon. Sauté until the bacon is cooked
and the onion is soft. Transfer the bacon and onion
to a bowl, using a slotted spoon.

Add the corned beef, beetroot, potatoes and
parsley. Season with salt and pepper and mix.

Heat the fat remaining in the pan, then add the
hash mixture. Level the surface with a knife and
press down lightly. Cook over a moderate heat for
15–20 minutes. Turn upside-down on to a plate to
serve. Serves 1.

Sausages and mash
500 Calories

200 g/7 oz potatoes, weighed peeled
60 ml/4 tablespoons skimmed milk
salt and pepper
2 large pork or beef sausages
125 g/4 oz frozen peas

Cook the potatoes in boiling water until tender.
Drain and mash with the skimmed milk. Season
with salt and pepper to taste. Meanwhile, cook the
sausages under a preheated grill until well done.
Cook the peas in enough boiling water to cover for
5 minutes, drain and serve with the sausages and
mash. Serves 1.

Chicken with jacket potato and corn
500 Calories

1 × 200 g/7 oz potato, scrubbed and pricked
1 × 275 g/10 oz chicken leg joint
125 g/4 oz sweetcorn, frozen or canned
15 ml/1 level tablespoon relish, any flavour

Bake the potato in its jacket in a preheated moderately hot oven (200°C/400°F, Gas Mark 6), for 50 to 60 minutes, until soft when pinched. Bake the chicken joint in a small dish beside the potato for the last 30 minutes. Remove the skin from the chicken and discard. Cook the frozen sweetcorn according to packet instructions or heat if canned. Serve with the potato, chicken and relish. Serves 1.

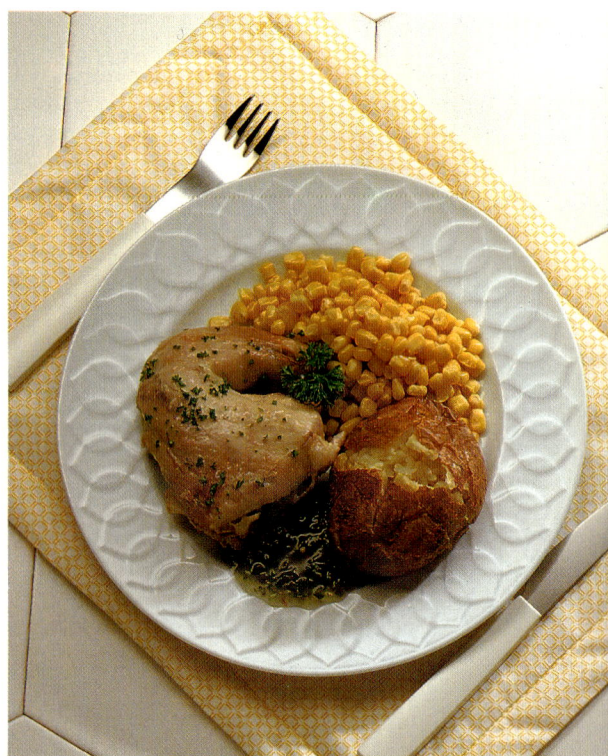

Beefburger and baked beans
500 Calories

1 large beefburger, 125 g/4 oz
1 × 40 g/1½ oz bap
1 × 150 g/5.3 oz can baked beans in tomato sauce
1 level tablespoon relish, any flavour, or tomato
   ketchup

Grill the burger well. Split the bap and toast the
cut sides. Heat the beans. Fill the bap with the
beefburger and relish and serve with the baked
beans. Serves 1.

BELOW LEFT: Chicken with jacket potato and corn.
BELOW: Beefburger with baked beans.

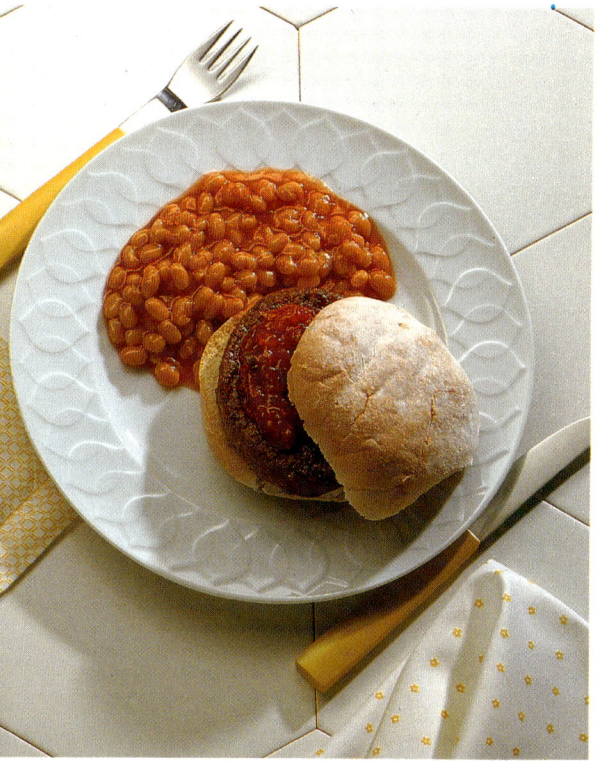

Egg, bacon and baked beans
500 Calories

2 rashers back bacon
1 × 227 g/8 oz can baked beans in tomato sauce
30 ml/2 tablespoons vegetable oil
1 egg, size 3
1 × 40 g/1½ oz slice wholemeal bread, toasted

Grill the bacon well. Put the baked beans in a saucepan to heat up. Heat the oil in a small frying pan and fry the egg. Drain well and discard any remaining fat. Serve the bacon and egg with the baked beans and the toast. Serves 1.

Eggs and chips
500 Calories

175 g/6 oz frozen grill chips or oven chips
30 ml/2 tablespoons vegetable oil
2 eggs, size 3
30 ml/2 level tablespoons tomato ketchup or
    brown sauce

Cook the chips according to packet instructions. Heat the oil in a small frying pan, fry the eggs and drain well. Discard any remaining fat. Serve with the chips and tomato ketchup or brown sauce. Serves 1.

Mixed grill with baked beans
500 Calories

1 × 50 g/2 oz beefburger
1 pork or beef chipolata sausage
100 g/3½ oz round bacon or ham steak
1 lamb's kidney, halved and cored
1 tomato, halved
1 × 225 g/8 oz can baked beans in tomato sauce

Place the burger, sausage, bacon steak and kidney under a preheated moderate grill and cook until well done, adding the tomato and cook for the last few minutes. Heat the baked beans in a saucepan and serve with the mixed grill. Serves 1.

Rump steak

500 Calories

1 × 200 g/7 oz potato, scrubbed and pricked
1 × 175 g/6 oz rump or sirloin steak, trimmed of
  excess fat
2 tomatoes, halved
125 g/4 oz button mushrooms
5 ml/1 level teaspoon made mustard

Bake the potato in its jacket in a preheated moderately hot oven (200°C/400°F, Gas Mark 6) for 50 to 60 minutes or until soft when pinched.

Cook the steak under a preheated grill until medium or well done. Add the tomatoes to the grill pan for the last 3–4 minutes of cooking. Poach the mushrooms in a little boiling salted water and drain. Serve the steak and vegetables with the mustard. Serves 1.

BELOW: Rump steak.

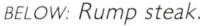

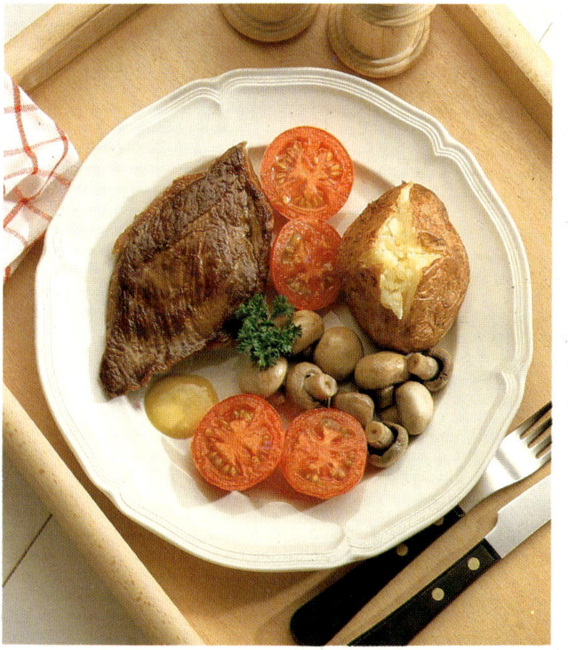

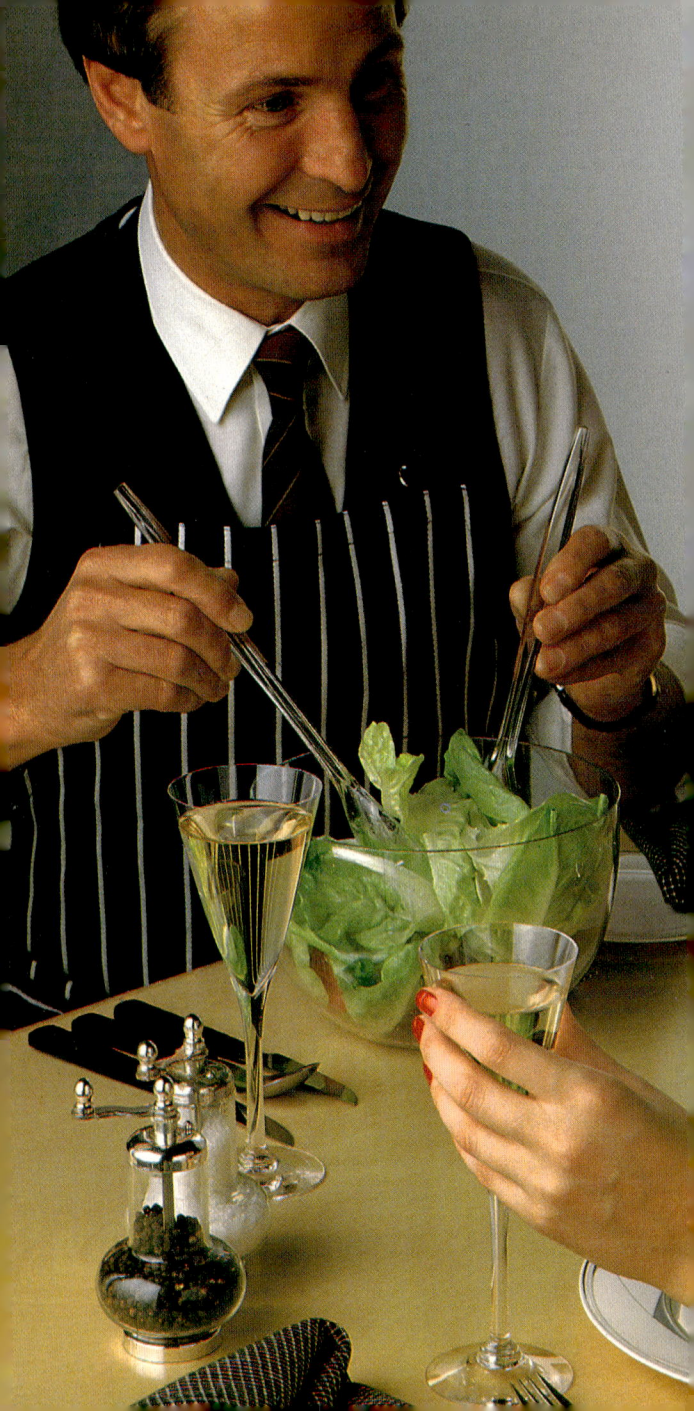

MAIN MEALS TO SHARE

There is no need to eat alone because you are trying to lose weight. All the main meals in this section serve 2, and can be doubled to serve 4.

Calorie cutters

★ It takes about twenty minutes for your brain to register that some food has reached your stomach, so eat slowly and you may eat less.
★ Fresh fruit makes a very low calorie start or finish to a meal. Try a slice of melon sprinkled with ginger.
★ Double cream contains 55 Calories per 15 ml tablespoon. In many instances half cream will serve equally well and will save you 35 Calories on the same quantity.

Lamb parcels with baked potatoes
500 Calories per portion

2 × 225 g/8 oz potatoes, scrubbed and pricked
½ small green or red pepper, cored, seeded and diced
2 spring onions, chopped
50 g/2 oz button mushrooms, chopped
1 small carrot, grated
10 ml/2 teaspoons soy sauce
salt and pepper
1 × 300 g/11 oz boneless lamb leg steak, trimmed of excess fat and halved
225 g/8 oz French beans or haricots verts, fresh or frozen

Bake the potatoes in their jackets in a preheated moderately hot oven (190°C/375°F, Gas Mark 5) for 1 hour or until soft when pinched.

Meanwhile, mix all the remaining vegetables, except the beans in a bowl and stir in the soy sauce. Season with salt and pepper.

Cut 2 squares of foil, each large enough to enclose half the meat and vegetables in a loose parcel. Divide half the vegetables between the foil squares and place a piece of lamb on top of each. Cover with the remaining vegetables. Wrap loosely, making sure that the edges are tightly sealed. Bake alongside the potatoes for 45 minutes. Cook the beans in boiling water until tender and serve with the lamb parcels and potatoes. Serves 2.

Goulash with noodles
500 Calories per portion

275 g/10 oz lean pork leg steaks or fillet,
   trimmed of excess fat and cubed
30 ml/2 level tablespoons flour
10 ml/2 level teaspoons paprika
5 ml/1 level teaspoon caraway seeds
salt and pepper

BELOW: Lamb parcels with baked potatoes, page 113.
BELOW RIGHT: Goulash with noodles.

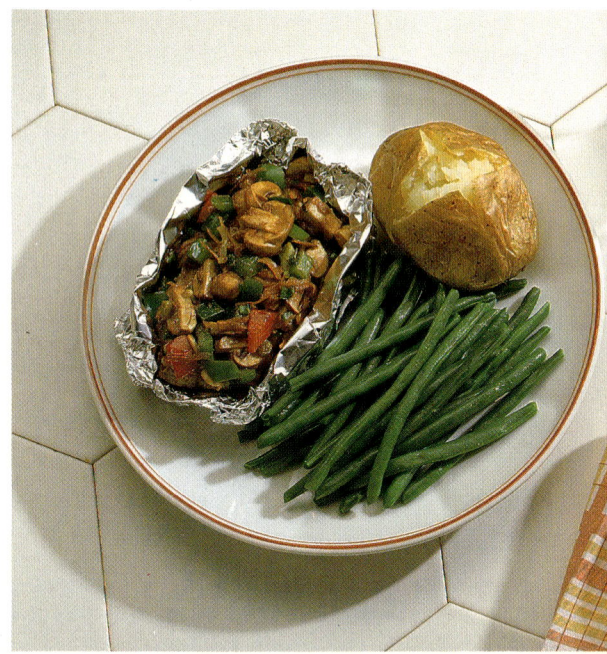

I small onion, chopped
$\frac{1}{2}$ green or red pepper, cored, seeded and sliced
I bouquet garni
$\frac{1}{2}$ chicken stock cube
15 ml/I level tablespoon tomato purée
225 ml/8 fl oz hot water
125 g/4 oz noodles
30 ml/2 level tablespoons soured cream (optional)

Place the pork in a casserole and sprinkle it with the flour, paprika and caraway seeds. Turn the meat so that all the pieces are coated. Season. Add the onion, pepper and bouquet garni.

Dissolve the stock cube and tomato purée in the hot water and pour over the meat and vegetables. Cover and cook in a preheated moderate oven (170°C/325°F, Gas Mark 3) for $1\frac{1}{4}$ hours.

Fifteen minutes before the end of cooking, boil the noodles. Drain and divide between 2 plates. Remove the bouquet garni, stir in the soured cream and serve on the noodles. Serves 2.

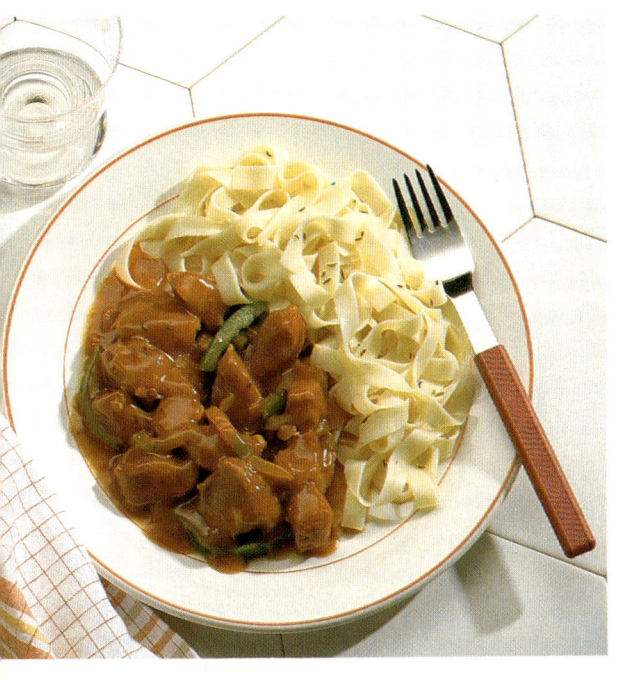

Shepherds pie and peas
500 Calories per portion

275 g/10 oz lean minced beef
15 ml/1 level tablespoon flour
1 small onion, finely chopped
10 ml/2 level teaspoons tomato purée
1.25 ml/$\frac{1}{4}$ level teaspoon mixed dried herbs
$\frac{1}{2}$ beef stock cube
120 ml/4 fl oz hot water
salt and pepper
450 g/1 lb potatoes, weighed peeled
90 ml/6 tablespoons skimmed milk
225 g/8 oz frozen peas

Brown the meat in a non-stick saucepan, then drain off and discard all the fat. Stir the flour into the meat with the onion, tomato purée and herbs. Turn into an ovenproof dish. Dissolve the stock cube in the water and add to the dish. Stir well. Season with salt and pepper and cover with a lid or foil. Cook in a preheated moderate oven (180°C/ 350°F, Gas Mark 4) for 40 minutes.

Meanwhile, boil the potatoes until tender. Drain and mash with the milk. Season with salt and pepper to taste and spread on top of the meat. Return to the oven for a further 20 minutes. Cook the peas in boiling water to cover until tender, drain and serve with the pie. Serves 2.

Trout with bacon
500 Calories per portion

350 g/12 oz potatoes, weighed peeled
25 g/1 oz very finely chopped onion
2 × 200 g/7 oz trout, defrosted if frozen
2 rashers streaky bacon, lightly grilled, cut into
    small strips
150 ml/$\frac{1}{4}$ pint dry cider
salt and pepper
10 ml/2 level teaspoons cornflour
30 ml/2 tablespoons cold water
225 g/8 oz frozen mixed vegetables

Cook the potatoes in plenty of boiling water. Meanwhile, place the onion in an ovenproof dish large enough to take the trout side by side. Season the insides of the trout and arrange in the dish. Scatter the bacon on top and pour in the cider. Cover the dish and cook in a preheated moderate oven (200°C/400°F, Gas Mark 6) for 20–30 minutes.

Transfer the cider carefully to a pan. Keep the fish warm. In a cup, blend the cornflour with the cold water. Stir into the cider and then bring to the boil, stirring all the time. Pour over the trout and keep warm. Cook the mixed vegetables in boiling water to cover, drain and serve with the trout and potatoes. Serves 2.

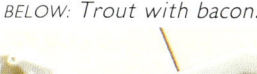

Calorie cutter

* It is important to measure spoonfuls carefully. A rounded tablespoon costs twice the calories of a level tablespoon and a heaped tablespoon costs three times as much.

BELOW: Trout with bacon.

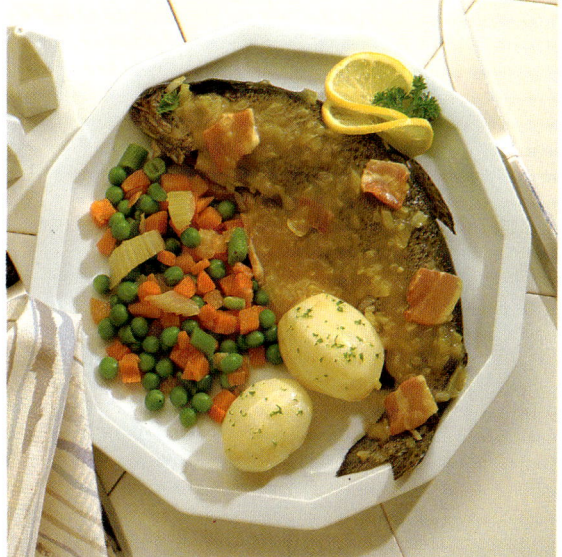

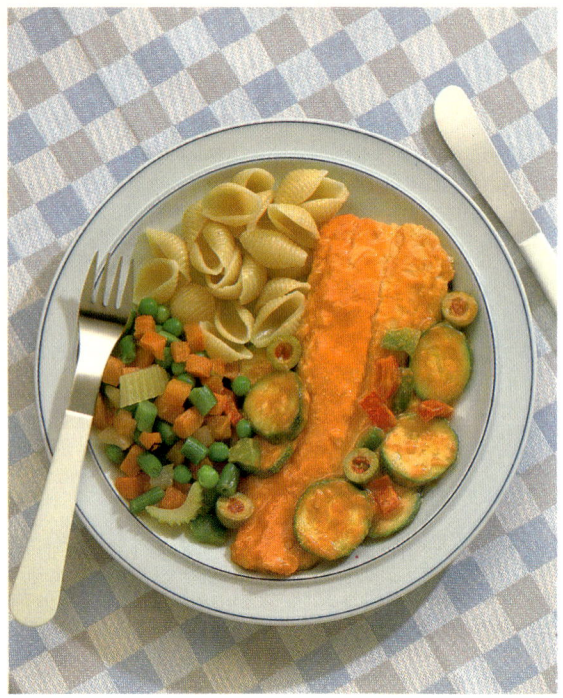

ABOVE: Fish Provençale.

Fish Provençale
500 Calories per portion

275 g/10 oz frozen cod, coley or haddock fillet
1 medium courgette, sliced
$\frac{1}{2}$ green or red pepper, cored, seeded and diced
4 stuffed olives, halved
1 clove garlic, crushed
1 × 140 g/4.9 oz can condensed cream of tomato soup
125 g/4 oz pasta shells or shapes
275 g/10 oz frozen mixed vegetables

Place the frozen fish fillets in an ovenproof dish in a single layer. Arrange the courgette, pepper and olives around the fish.

Stir the garlic into the undiluted soup. Spread over the fish and vegetables. Do not season – the soup will contain seasoning enough. Cover with a lid or foil and cook in a preheated moderately hot oven (200°C/400°F, Gas Mark 6) for 35 minutes or until the fish flakes easily when touched with a fork. Cook the pasta and the mixed vegetables in separate saucepans of boiling water, drain and serve with the fish. Serves 2.

Ginger chicken with nutty pilaf
500 Calories per portion

2 × 275 g/10 oz chicken leg joints, skinned and
    trimmed of fat
5 ml/1 level teaspoon butter or margarine
1.25 ml/$\frac{1}{4}$ level teaspoon ground ginger
300 ml/$\frac{1}{2}$ pint low-calorie ginger ale
salt and pepper
75 g/3 oz long-grain white rice
30 ml/2 level tablespoons currants
250 ml/8 fl oz boiling water
125 g/4 oz frozen peas
15 ml/1 level tablespoon cornflour, blended with
    30 ml/2 tablespoons cold water
25 g/1 oz hazelnuts, toasted

Place the chicken in a casserole. Melt the butter in a small saucepan and stir in the ground ginger. Add the ginger ale and season with salt and pepper. Pour over the chicken. Cover and set aside.

Place the rice and currants in another casserole. Pour in the boiling water, season with salt and pepper and cover. Place both casseroles in a preheated moderate oven (180°C/350°F, Gas Mark 4) and bake for 30 minutes. Remove both casseroles from the oven. Mix the peas with the rice and stir the cornflour mixture into the chicken casserole. Return both casseroles to the oven and cook for a further 15 minutes.

Stir the hazelnuts into the rice just before serving it with the chicken. Serves 2.

Beef stew with dumplings
500 Calories per portion

250 g/9 oz lean stewing steak, trimmed of all
    visible fat and cubed
15 ml/1 level tablespoon cornflour
1 medium onion, sliced
75 g/3 oz carrots, sliced
1 bouquet garni
1 beef stock cube
275 ml/$\frac{1}{2}$ pint hot water
225 g/8 oz can butter beans, drained
Dumplings:
50 g/2 oz self-raising flour
25 g/1 oz shredded suet
pinch of salt

Place the meat in a casserole. Sprinkle on the
cornflour and mix well so that all the pieces of meat
are coated. Add the onion and carrots with the
bouquet garni. Dissolve the stock cube in the
water and pour over the meat and vegetables.
Cover the dish and cook in a preheated moderate
oven (150°C/300°F/Gas Mark 2) for $2\frac{1}{2}$ hours.
    Stir the beans into the casserole. For the dump-
lings, place the flour in a bowl and mix with the suet
and salt. Add enough water to make a firm dough
and divide into 4. Shape into balls and place on the
casserole. Return to the oven and cook covered for
10 minutes, then uncovered for 10 minutes more.
Remove the bouquet garni and serve. Serves 2.

Chinese-style chicken breasts
500 Calories per portion

2 × 225 g/8 oz part-boned chicken breasts,
    skinned
30 ml/2 tablespoons light soy sauce
15 ml/1 tablespoon clear honey
5 ml/1 level teaspoon Chinese five spice powder
1.25 ml/$\frac{1}{4}$ level teaspoon ground ginger
salt and pepper
75 g/3 oz brown or white long-grain rice
15 ml/1 tablespoon vegetable oil
225 g/8 oz frozen stir-fry vegetables

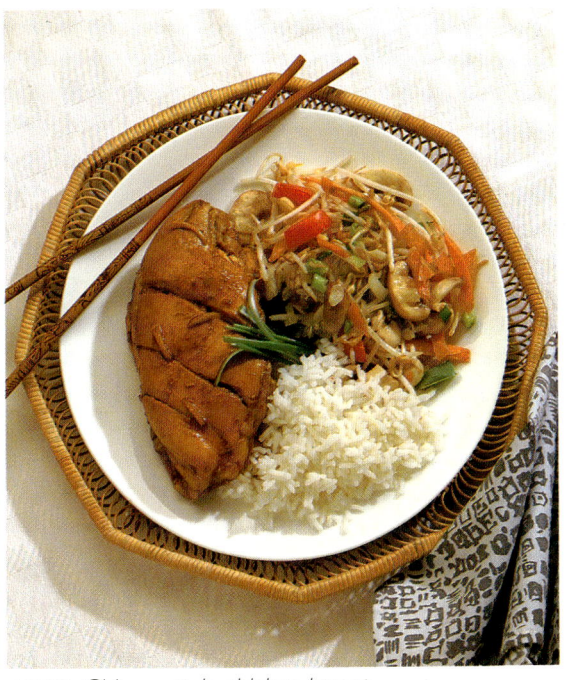

ABOVE: Chinese-style chicken breast.

Make 3 deep cuts in the flesh of each chicken breast. Place in an ovenproof dish. In a bowl, mix together the soy sauce, honey, five spice powder and ginger. Add salt and pepper to taste. Spoon over the chicken breasts and turn them over so that they are completely coated in the marinade. Cover and refrigerate for 4 to 12 hours, turning once or twice.

Bake in a preheated moderate oven (180°C/ 350°F, Gas Mark 4) for 45 minutes. Meanwhile cook the rice in plenty of boiling water until tender. Drain and keep warm. Heat the oil in a non-stick frying pan or wok, then stir-fry the frozen vegetables for 4 minutes. Serve with the chicken breasts and rice. Serves 2.

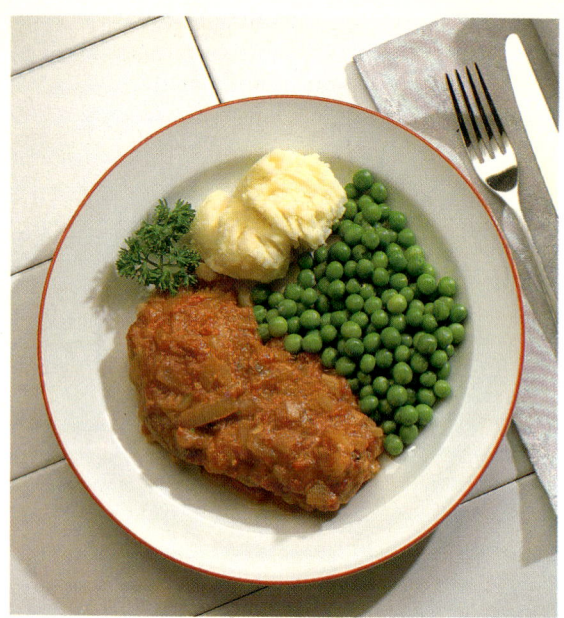

ABOVE: *Swiss steak.*

Swiss steak
500 Calories per portion

20 ml/4 level teaspoons flour
salt and pepper
350 g/12 oz lean braising steak, trimmed of
    excess fat and halved
1 small onion, roughly chopped
1 small clove garlic, crushed
1 × 227 g/8 oz can tomatoes, roughly chopped
5 ml/1 level teaspoon tomato purée
45 ml/3 tablespoons water
1 small bay leaf
400 g/14 oz potatoes, weighed peeled
90 ml/6 tablespoons skimmed milk (optional)
225 g/8 oz frozen peas

Place the flour in a plastic bag and season with salt
and pepper. Add the meat and shake until all the
surfaces are coated. Place in a casserole with the

excess flour. Add the onion, garlic and the tomatoes with their juice. Stir in the tomato purée, water and bay leaf and cover.

Cook in a preheated cool oven (150°C/300°F, Gas Mark 2) for 3 hours. Thirty minutes before the end of cooking, boil the potatoes. Drain and if old, mash with the milk. If new, leave whole. Cook the peas in boiling water until tender and drain. Remove the bay leaf from the steak and serve with the peas and potatoes. Serves 2.

Fish and broccoli in cheese sauce
500 Calories per portion

225 g/8 oz broccoli, fresh or frozen
350 g/12 oz cod or haddock fillet
150 ml/$\frac{1}{4}$ pint skimmed milk
salt and pepper
350 g/12 oz potatoes, weighed peeled
225 g/8 oz carrots, fresh or frozen
15 g/$\frac{1}{2}$ oz low-fat spread
15 g/$\frac{1}{2}$ oz flour
50 g/2 oz Edam cheese, grated
30 ml/2 level tablespoons fresh breadcrumbs

Cook the broccoli in a saucepan of boiling water until just tender. Drain and arrange on the base of an ovenproof dish.

Meanwhile, place the fish and milk in a shallow, wide-based pan. Season, then cover and simmer gently until the fish flakes easily when touched with a fork – about 5 to 10 minutes. Reserving the milk in the pan, transfer the fish to the ovenproof dish, using a slotted spoon, and keep it warm. In separate pans, boil the potatoes and carrots until tender.

Melt the low-fat spread in a small pan. Stir in the flour. Add the reserved milk and bring to the boil, whisking all the time. Reduce the heat and simmer, stirring, for 1 minute. Stir in $\frac{2}{3}$ of the cheese. Pour the cheese sauce over the fish and sprinkle the remaining cheese and the breadcrumbs on top. Place under a preheated grill until the top starts to brown. Serve with the drained potatoes and carrots. Serves 2.

INDEX

ACKNOWLEDGEMENTS
The publishers would like to thank Duncan
McNicol for providing all the photographs
except:
Zefa Picture Library (UK) Ltd p. 13.

0135